ANCIENT EGYPT AND MODERN PSYCHOTHERAPY

In *Ancient Egypt and Modern Psychotherapy*, Todd Hayen explores what the spiritual concepts of the enigmatic ancient Egyptians can teach us about our own modern psyches and the pursuit of a meaningful life.

Hayen examines the ancient Egyptians' possession of a concept contemporary academics have labeled "consciousness of the heart": an innate knowledge of the entirety of the universe. While all human beings possess this consciousness of the heart, our modern culture has largely lost the ability to tap into this inborn knowledge. By examining the material accomplishments of ancient Egypt, and how the Egyptians' seemingly deeper awareness of their inner world created a harmonious outer world, we can begin to understand how modern psychotherapy, through a Jungian perspective, could be instrumental in achieving a more profound and meaningful personal experience of life.

Ancient Egypt and Modern Psychotherapy will be insightful reading for analytical psychologists in practice and in training, Jungian psychotherapists and psychologists, and academics and students of Jungian and post-Jungian studies and ancient spirituality.

Todd Hayen is a psychotherapist in private practice in Toronto, Canada. He received his Ph.D. from Pacifica Graduate Institute in Santa Barbara in depth psychology with an emphasis on psychotherapy.

"Todd Hayen's book does what all good, creative scholarship does: it opens our minds to new ways of seeing something we thought we already knew. But it does more than this: it shows how we today can benefit from exploring the remarkable 'sacred science' of ancient Egypt. We need not 'walk like an Egyptian' to profit from understanding how they did, and their insights into the much-neglected soul seem to me to present better ways of healing our own fractured psyche than any amount of modern pharmacology. Hayen does not solve the 'mysteries of Egypt;' he invites us to share with him his evident passion for embracing them. The first step in any psychotherapy is taking our inner world seriously. The reader of this book soon sees that Hayen does."

Gary Lachman, associate professor in Transformative Studies at the California Institute of Integral Studies, USA and author of *The Secret Teachers of the Western World*

"Despite the fact that Todd Hayen draws from a very ancient culture, his views of modern psychotherapy are fresh and insightful. He confronts us with the shadow of modern society—materialism and an accompanying empirical science—that robs us of a vital connection to soul. By pointing out that the locus of intelligence has moved from the heart to the head, he recalls the sacred science of ancient Egypt where the heart was the threshold to the soul. As a psychotherapist, Todd knows first-hand the wounds suffered by this dislocation, and presents us with a new marriage between a sacred sensibility to what really matters in life, and how to revive the neglected soul in therapy. Anyone interested in this ancient wisdom tradition and who longs to 'wake up' to the splendor that lies hidden amidst the turmoil of modern society is advised not only to read this book but alchemically bring its words to life!"

Thom F. Cavalli, Ph.D., psychologist and author of *Embodying Osiris* and *Alchemical Psychology: Old Recipes for Living in a New World*

"A major theme of *Ancient Egypt and Modern Psychotherapy: Sacred Science and the Search for Soul* is that the psyche of an individual has a direct influence on the material world that individual inhabits. In this courageous, well documented, and heartfelt book, the talented composer and depth psychologist Dr. Todd Hayen draws from his personal experiences as well as his research into the consciousness of ancient Egypt to illustrate his concern with the lack of soul in our modern materialistic and rationalistic paradigm, a concern that he places squarely in the depth psychological tradition stemming from C.G. Jung, particularly Jung's research into the relationship between psyche and matter. The mysterious architectural achievements of the ancient Egyptians open the door to a wide-ranging survey of Hayen's metaphysical and parapsychological interests, and to a compelling reflection on what a sacred science might look like today, especially in the context of psychotherapy. At the core of this book is a meditation on the mystery of the relationship between inner and outer, psyche and matter, and subjectivity and objectivity that opens the reader's mind to new thoughts and intuitions concerning both ancient and contemporary experiences of the interconnections between the seen and unseen worlds."

Thomas Elsner, J.D., M.A., Jungian analyst, Faculty Pacifica Graduate Institute, USA

ANCIENT EGYPT AND MODERN PSYCHOTHERAPY

Sacred Science and the Search for Soul

Todd Hayen

Routledge
Taylor & Francis Group
LONDON AND NEW YORK

First published 2017
by Routledge
2 Park Square, Milton Park, Abingdon, Oxon OX14 4RN

and by Routledge
605 Third Avenue, New York, NY 10017

Routledge is an imprint of the Taylor & Francis Group, an informa business

British Library Cataloguing in Publication Data
A catalogue record for this book is available from the British Library

Library of Congress Cataloging in Publication Data
Names: Hayen, Todd, author.
Title: Ancient Egypt and modern psychotherapy : sacred science and the search for soul / Todd Hayen.
Description: Abingdon, Oxon ; New York, NY : Routledge, 2017. | Includes bibliographical references.
Identifiers: LCCN 2016032187 | ISBN 9781138122178 (hbk. : alk. paper) | ISBN 9781138122185 (pbk. : alk. paper) | ISBN 9781315650593 (ebk.)
Subjects: | MESH: Psychotherapy | Psychoanalytic Theory | Jungian Theory | Mind-Body Relations, Metaphysical | Psychology, Comparative | History, Ancient | Egypt
Classification: LCC RC480.5 | NLM WM 420 | DDC 616.89/14—dc23
LC record available at https://lccn.loc.gov/2016032187

ISBN: 978-1-138-12217-8 (hbk)
ISBN: 978-1-138-12218-5 (pbk)
ISBN: 978-1-315-65059-3 (ebk)

Typeset in Bembo
by Swales & Willis Ltd, Exeter, Devon, UK

For Cindy

CONTENTS

ACKNOWLEDGMENTS

I offer thanks to the ancient Egyptians for their unsurpassed soulfulness and the inspiration they stirred in me during their frequent visits into my imaginal space.

Among the scholars and scientists who furthered my understanding of the mysteries of Egypt, appreciation goes to Christopher Dunn for his exacting work in the deserts of Egypt, to Robert Schoch for his incredible discoveries regarding the age of the Sphinx, to Gary Lachman for his astonishing scholarship and inquisitive mind, to Stephen Braude for his bravery in stepping out on a limb, and to R. A. Schwaller de Lubicz for his remarkable insight and ability to see the ancient Egyptians in a way no one before him could see. Gratitude also goes to Jeremy Naydler, a consummate scholar and source of inspiration.

I am deeply indebted to Tom Elsner for his belief in my work and in me. Thanks to Mike Denney and Robin van Löben Sels, who were the first to review these pages, and to Jan Freya as well for her impeccable work as my editor.

I extend thanks to my family: to my two sisters, Charla and Tara, for their unending emotional and creative support, and to my stepfather, Harold Herman, for being a father to me during most of my later childhood years and teaching me about purpose and value in creative pursuits. Deep gratitude goes to my late wife Janice, who encouraged me many years ago to embark on this academic and spiritual journey and whose love and support nurtured me through the first part of my life; to my mother, for her soulful creative spark, which lit the way for me as an artist; and last but not least, to my wife Cindy, whose love, dedication, and belief in me casts a bright, burning illumination onto many dark and murky shadows.

Material from the film *Matter of Heart* is included here by kind permission of the C. G. Jung Institute of Los Angeles.

Desert Dream by Michael Parkes is included here by kind permission of Michael and Maria Parkes.

INTRODUCTION

Egypt—the name of this enigmatic place can be alluring to those who have even scant knowledge of its history and cosmology. In ancient times, the word that was used to describe the name of the land now known as Egypt was *Kemi* or *Kemit*, which meant "black land," due to the unusual richness of the soil nurtured by the yearly inundation of the Nile. The familiar modern designation comes to us through several permutations, beginning with the Greek *Aiguptos*, which is believed to be a variant of the Egyptian *Hat-kuptah*: "Temple of the *Ka* of Ptah." What is it about this place that holds such magic and mystery for so many that have experienced it either directly, through study and travel, or through a more subjective route including dreams and literary or imagined fantasy?

Perhaps we are attracted to the thirst-quenching oasis of spiritual enlightenment and are drawn to the awareness the ancient Egyptians possessed about the true nature of reality—a wholeness of being, infusing animated life into all things physical and nonphysical. The ancient Egyptians believed that the material world as well as the imaginal inner world was infused with spirit and spirits. They believed in a wholly integrated reality, which included the physical forms of nature as well as the unseen images, gods, goddesses, powers, symbols, and meanings that go beyond a rational, intellectual comprehension to present a harmonized inner and outer perception of reality.

This book utilizes a method of inquiry that keeps soul in mind while interpreting the resources used to investigate the spiritual substance of important concepts such as the psyche-to-matter problem (discussed in Chapter 4) and the loss of an awareness of soul in a modern materialist paradigm. This book explores how ancient Egyptian sacred science relates to the variety of ways in which humankind has defined soul and spirit and how this ancient Egyptian way of being could be integrated in modern modalities of science, medicine, and, most significantly, the practice of psychotherapy. From a conventional perspective, psychotherapy is presently considered from a largely materialistic viewpoint, with little or no regard for the unseen and immeasurable presence of soul. This book examines how the integration of the principles and practices of Egyptian sacred science would impact today's understanding of reality and our own individual management of our lives.

The general consensus among mainstream Egyptologists is that the First Dynastic Kingdom of ancient Egypt began approximately 5,000 years ago. Alternative historians believe the civilization may be much older than that. The last kingdom of ancient Egypt ended with the rein of Cleopatra VII and the Ptolemaic–Greek period in approximately 30 BCE. For the following 1,760 years the great temples and structures of a 3,000-year-old grand civilization sank slowly into the sands of Northeastern Africa. Into the underworld Egypt descended, sinking deeper and deeper, through the Roman conquests and the subsequent Arab invasions and occupation, all but disappearing as the centuries marched on. The Napoleonic campaign into Egypt in 1798 can be seen as a symbol of Egypt's emergence from the underworld—lifting her once proud and noble presence from the sands of the desert, signifying the end of this particular cycle in human history. After Napoleon began to brush the sand away from her treasures and the secrets of the Rosetta Stone were finally revealed, ancient Egypt began once again to show her brilliance after her journey through the shadowy underworld of obscurity and faded memory. She now brings an awareness of her secrets to the modern world and sparks a keen desire from its current diverse occupants to learn her ancient, mysterious, and sacred ways.

This book also takes the reader on a journey into the underworld of transformation, starting with descriptions of the miracles found in ancient Egypt, which could only have been executed with an understanding unknown to modern sensibilities; through a brief explanation of possible mechanisms for the implementation of these wonders; and finally into possible means of integrating into our own modern psyches the cosmology of the ancient Egyptians. This book is not about historical Egypt per se—you will not find histories of the Pharaohs, descriptions of the Egyptian gods, or details of the military campaigns in the ancient Middle East. You also will not find a concise methodology for integrating an Egyptian way of being with modern psychotherapy, although suggestions as to how to implement this special and unique perspective are certainly proposed. It is not necessary for us to become replicas of the ancient Egyptians in ritual, look, and style, to benefit from the concepts of their sacred science or to apply an ancient way of relating to the universe through similar rituals and customs. The Egyptian way can be applied in our modern culture by our adaptation and immersion in the fundamentals the ancients expressed in their cosmology.

Mainstream Egyptology is a noble pursuit, like all serious study founded on the spirit of curiosity and the quest for knowledge. Most Egyptologists are passionate and dedicated scholars, striving to understand an enigmatic people who lived, worked, and worshipped their gods a very long time ago. They do, however, work within the confines of a materialist paradigm and cannot, or do not care to, expand their speculations and conclusions to include more metaphysical and nonmaterial perceptions. It is not my intention to disparage their work in any way but rather to suggest opening a few doors into what has been forbidden territory in order to observe these mysteries illuminated by a different quality of light.

In addition, I have not intended to paint a picture of a perfect ancient Egyptian culture. There is ample evidence of dysfunctional, destructive, and unenlightened behavior among the Egyptians. Murder, manipulation, xenophobia, genocide, and even drunkenness and spousal abuse seem to have been common occurrences among the peoples of this ancient culture. Medical maladies, disease, and parasites also clearly occupied the ancient Egyptian world. Why would a civilization that had the power and insight and, quite possibly, a metaphysical energy to create astounding monuments, statuary, and scientific accomplishments suffer such obvious human deficiencies? This is an important question, but I will not attempt to answer it. Much that we know of Egyptian life beyond the religious temple texts and other writing comes from careful and informed speculation. Interpretations are generally flavored by an understanding of human behavior based on more modern cultures, including our current one, as models of what human beings typically do, think, and dream. This approach is certainly a rational one and fits well within the scientific method of inquiry. It cannot, however, be expected to tell the whole story. What if the ancient Egyptians were little like us or other civilizations that emerged after them? It stands to reason that they were essentially the same, in basic psychological and physical ways, as other human beings—but what if they were not? I leave this question unanswered as well and invite readers to continue their own personal research to shed more light on this enigmatic culture.

We live in perilous times. The planet has never been in such a state of chaos and dysfunction, which can surely be seen as a reflection of the chaos and dysfunction within the individual psyches of the planet's human inhabitants. On a global level we see the depletion of the earth's resources and the insane human destruction of its physical structure through deforestation, mineral mining, nuclear and chemical pollution, and the extraction of oil as well as a wanton disregard for the other living creatures that share the planet with us through overfishing, habitat destruction, and factory farming. Not only is our physical environment being systematically destroyed, but the very essence of our being as spiritual entities is being challenged. Through materialism, consumerism, and disregard for the whole of reality—which includes spirit and the inner world of image and symbol as well as the physical world of matter—we have, as a collective, lost sight of our soul. Reintegration with a deeper and more complete consciousness—a consciousness of the heart coupled with the prevailing consciousness of the intellect—may be the only hope we have for saving our planet and ourselves. This endeavor begins with an inner journey—a journey into our own psyches to rediscover our hidden and thirsty souls.

1

WHY ANCIENT EGYPT?

The small six-seater tour bus bounced noisily along the washboard road as we approached the Serapeum excavation in the northwestern part of Egypt's Saqqara, the burial site for the sacred Apis bulls. Nothing could be seen ahead of us but an off-white blanket of sizzling sand almost too bright to look at. The undulating shimmer of desert heat that sat seemingly a foot or so off the desert's surface was just as much felt as seen. The heat seemed to permeate everything and rippled through our bodies just as it rippled across the desert creating the glowing mirages often seen dancing on the barren landscape.

At the time of our visit in 1993 the Serapeum was not a usual tourist attraction, and it took some coercion, and a few Egyptian pounds, to get our tour guide to include it on our final day of adventure in Egypt. Our small group of intrepid travelers included my first wife Janice, me, and our friends Frank and Tracey, who had decided to tag along when we announced one evening over dinner that we had finally decided to do something really crazy and travel to Egypt. We all worked together in the film music business in Hollywood, and after many years of having our noses glued to the grindstone of endless work and focus on career, we felt that we needed to get completely off the grid, at least for a moment. "Let's do something really exotic!" I proclaimed, after a particularly exhausting day of back-to-back recording sessions. "Let's go to Egypt!" Much to my surprise, Janice agreed, after what seemed to be negligible consideration. Soon we were sharing the news with our friends who were equally ensconced in the mind-numbing pursuit of "the next gig" in the jungles of the Hollywood movie industry. Before any of us could change our minds, the plans for the trip were finalized, and we found ourselves in one of the most exotic and intriguing places on earth.

The little dilapidated bus skittered to a halt on the loose sand and gravel of the small parking area, after what seemed to be hours of bumpy driving in the expansive Egyptian nowhere-land. The entrance to the attraction looked to be only a moderate pile of rocks placed a few steps away from the parking lot. There was a little sign stuck in the sand at the far edge of the pile that read in both Arabic and English: *Serapeum*. Although more than likely untrue, one got the impression that the hand-lettered placards that accompanied all Egyptian tourist attractions were created during the Victorian time of French- and English-dominated Egyptology more than 150 years ago. We all stepped out of the bus and brushed off the ubiquitous sand that seeped into any space, enclosed or not, and headed for the entrance to the Serapeum, which consisted of an unwieldy-looking set of makeshift stairs that plunged steeply into the dark, but ultimately cooler, recesses of subterranean Egypt.

The Serapeum, we were told by our tour guide, is an underground labyrinth of small chambers that each held a large granite sarcophagus presumably intended to hold the mummified remains of the Apis bull. Twenty-four such sarcophagi exist at this site. Although undeniably interesting, such a place did not seem uniquely mysterious before we actually were in it, other than what is characteristically felt to be mysterious regarding ancient Egypt's culture and customs in general.

We unsteadily descended the stairs and, after several minutes of precarious footwork, entered into the cavernous anteroom of the Serapeum itself and stopped to catch our breath. We stood huddled in a small group looking down an adjacent corridor lit by a string of old, clear light bulbs suspended from the ceiling by twisted, rusting wire ties. A large black granite box about the size of a small car stood in the narrow passage almost blocking it—its presence there never adequately explained by our tour guide. The oppressive nature of the space was palpable, and although a dozen or so degrees cooler than the desert floor where we had left the bus, the air was hot and fetid. Our physical senses registered and measured all of these things as best they could, but something else was being felt in that space. For me, it was a sense of magic, mystery, and profundity that I can in no way adequately describe in words. I felt I was in a sacred space, which contained sacred things with a sacred intent.

We walked down the dim corridor, the flickering bulbs overhead, passing small largely unlit chambers, which lined each side of the passageway. Most of them were empty, but within several were clones of the large granite box we had seen in the antechamber. We were guided into one of these rooms, and although the space was small, we all managed to place ourselves in some sort of order around the large, unearthly stone presence placed in the center of the room. One thing that struck me as intriguing as I visited each site in Egypt was how its description as presented in books and other literature paled in comparison to the actual experience of seeing, in front of oneself with one's own eyes, the monument, temple, or artifact that had been described. The Serapeum was no exception.

As if all of us in the room were being channeled the same question simultaneously, each of us looked around at our surroundings and the 80-ton granite box in front of us and said, "How did this get in here?" I would suppose that most visitors asked the same question, and for a question that undoubtedly was asked hundreds of times, the tour guide had no answer.

This was a question for me that simply wouldn't go away. I kept looking at the entrance, the large box—which measured approximately 13 feet long, 7½ feet wide, and 10 feet high—as well as the narrow walkway around it, which was about 5 feet wide from the edge of the sarcophagus to the stone-and-dirt wall of the enclosing room, and wondering how it had all occurred. The ceiling was cut from the rock and dirt as well, so there was no possibility of lowering the box into the space. At that time, I had no knowledge of the work of the machining engineer Christopher Dunn, who had conducted preliminary research in Egypt regarding ancient technology and engineering techniques. Dunn, who visited the Serapeum a few years after our visit to measure production tolerances on the granite boxes, determined that the accuracy of construction on the sarcophagi was simply too precise to reason, with their supposed purpose and nature of creation. This information, if I had had it at the time, would have unquestionably added to the mystery.

What, exactly, were we looking at? And how and why was it there?

The final veil of mystery regarding this enchanting place lightly fell over my awareness, and my engulfment by its wonder was complete. Was this merely a matter of highly advanced materialist engineering and technique, or did it include in its making something nonmaterial—some sort of mysterious and ineffable power—that was not considered at all by modern archeologists and scientists in their efforts to explain? Several alternative theories suggest that many of these artifacts and ancient sites predate dynastic Egypt and were actually inherited by the Egyptians and utilized in their religion and culture. More mainstream researchers, however, have insisted that these things are purely Egyptian but obviously are beyond our current, conventional view of the ancient Egyptians' abilities, technology, and scientific acumen.

After several minutes of further exploration and discovery, we all crawled out of the hole in the desert and returned to our wobbly tour bus. No one said much during the long drive back to civilization. The tour guide unwrapped a stick of gum and, after carefully folding it in half, put it in his mouth and began chewing. He looked out the window at the passing sameness of desert sand, seeming to be completely unconcerned about the mystery that still lay guarded and unanswered in the dark tunnels of the Serapeum. I gazed out the window as well and considered how difficult it seems to be to understand something that is so foreign, based on things with which I am familiar. After the initial shock of being faced with an impossibility that sits squarely in front of me, I tend to allow it to meld in with the rest of my internal unknowns—like the dog who looks up at a hot air balloon for the first time in amazement and confusion but quickly takes the position that it simply does not matter. I shook off the compulsion and was determined not to allow the excitement and intrigue of this experience to fade away. This land held secrets I wanted to explore.

Seeing first hand the marvels of Egypt in her art, architecture, engineering, and spiritual perspective of life and death during that first trip, I was continuously in awe of the accomplishments of this historically primitive culture. It was difficult to comprehend the feats accomplished here by a civilization that at the time of the supposed construction of the pyramids had not yet adopted the use of wheeled carts. Also in the Saqqara, at the mortuary temple, I stood in front of massive stones, which I had been informed were between 60 and 200 tons in weight, perched high above the desert floor atop other equally massive stones. I could not accept, in all of my objective reasoning, the curt and precise explanation that modern mainstream Egyptologists have given as to how these structures were engineered and constructed. It simply belied reason. Most other researchers intrigued by such phenomena look for the material means of their manifestation, often proclaiming sensational theories involving alien technology or tools and devices with laser-precision capabilities that have been lost to antiquity. My thoughts instead went to the potential powers of the mind. I pondered a nonmaterial solution—something more magical and, clearly, more metaphysical.

As I left the desert lands behind after our 1993 ten-day tour, I felt even more bewildered by Egypt's mysteries. Stepping out onto the tarmac at the Cairo airport to board our return flight to the United States, I filled my lungs with the dry Egyptian heat of early morning, just as the sun was beginning to ascend from its nightly transformative journey through the underworld. I felt as if I was leaving my real home in a certain sense. Many people in past-life regression therapy have described Egypt as the location of one of their distant early lives. Considering the overall effect this place had on my psyche, I possibly could have been one of them. I took in a deep breath and felt a familiar warmth in my lungs, as the hot air of *Kemit* filled my soul with awareness, energy, and life.

The ensuing years after this initial visit were personally difficult for me, as my wife of 28 years fell ill to cancer and, after a noble confrontation with the disease, succumbed to it four years after her diagnosis. Six years after her death, I fell in love with a woman I had met while attending graduate school, and soon after our initial meeting, we decided to share a trip to Egypt. This time I was a bit more prepared for what I experienced, at least from an objective, scientific point of view—I don't think I could ever have prepared enough for the spiritual experience I was sure to encounter. During the years between visits, I had become an amateur student of Egyptology—but not conventional Egyptology. I favored an alternative perspective. As odd as it sounds, the esoteric theories regarding the design and building of the many amazing structures in Egypt simply seemed more rational to me. Theories abound regarding the techniques actually utilized to build the pyramids, the temple structures, and the obelisks, and to perform the dozens of other seemingly impossible tasks the ancient Egyptians obviously accomplished. Some of these theories are comprehensible and seem rational and coherent, and a seemingly equal number do not.

Once I had discarded much of the conventional thought surrounding these construction methods due to their obvious physical problems, I had a much more plausible idea of how things had to have been done. Or did I? The plausible *how* I was now faced with defining was not explainable by our current known science. Regardless of the actual mechanism used (whether it fit within the confines of

Newtonian laws of physics or not), there seemed to be something clearly missing from most of these more esoteric formulations. It didn't seem to me to be so important to know the physical mechanism whereby these accomplishments came to be in the physical world. What did seem important was the human consciousness behind the mechanism, if there even was physical mechanism per se.

Most theories of Egyptian construction and execution endeavor to explain how something may have been accomplished physically—whether it be a conventional procedure such as building a ramp beside a pyramid structure to pull large stones up to their final position or an unconventional methodology involving antigravity devices and techniques. Both of these procedures, albeit radically different in their perspectives, still fall within a cause-and-effect paradigm: one, the more conventional, stays within the confining laws of our current known science; the other relies on something unseen and yet undiscovered (assuming it is even discoverable) and contradictory to our current understanding of how things are in a materially based universe.

What I was looking for was a radically different perspective. I struggled with this conundrum for quite some time until I discovered the works of two prominent authors and researchers on ancient Egypt. One was Robert Bauval (1999), who says, in his seminal book on the mysteries of Egypt, *Secret Chamber: The Quest for the Hall of Records*:

> Egyptology is not a "science," it is a *sacred science*. The Great Pyramid is not only an engineering structure conforming to clear geometrical rules, but a sacred temple of initiation into the mysteries of cosmic existence. To be sure, the ancient architect–priests used a geometrical canon to design their monuments, but this canon was an intrinsic part of the sacred science of initiation. Geometry was sacred. Art was sacred. Architecture was sacred. Hieroglyphs were sacred. Astronomy was sacred. They were all part and parcel of a sacred science taught to high initiates in the temple. The mind of man, which they deemed the most sacred thing of all creation, was to be made adept to this science or knowledge in order to find God. (pp. 53–54)

Bauval presents in this statement what I believe to be the true fundamental nature of the ancient Egyptian culture. In our current post-Enlightenment, materialist paradigm, the *meaning* of physical expression other than art is to be found through objective measurement: height, length, weight, precision, and functionality. Indeed, even art is measured through the senses. In this materialist paradigm, music is of no use if it cannot be heard with the ears, as well as painting, sculpture, and architecture being useless if they cannot be seen and thus quantified by sight. Bauval points out that there may have been another nonobjective, nonmaterial value present in Egyptian creative efforts—that being its sacredness in execution and presentation.

In the preceding pages of his book, Bauval (1999) recounts a description his brother read at a gathering of Egypt enthusiasts of hunting a certain type of

Egyptian bird that his brother, as a young boy growing up in Egypt, used to hunt and trap. Bauval describes his brother as a professional architect adept at the ancient teachings of sacred architecture. His reading went, in part, as follows:

> There is a small bird, a type of wagtail, known to the Egyptians as Abu Deil, "Father of Tails," which comes from Central Africa. Each year, in late September, this bird migrates north to the Egyptian shore of the Mediterranean. . . . Late September is, of course, the time of the autumn equinox, when the sky is clear and the air very still. The waters of the Nile are receding after the flood period in August, and there is a feeling of renewal of the vegetation and the thick and rich alluvial soil of the Nile Valley. The Abu Deil appears, as if by magic, at dawn, with the equinoctial sun rising due east. It likes the open desert, perching always on small rocks, watching, and communicating with the environment with the constant wagging of its tail. (p. 50)

The wagtail appears as a common occurrence in the form of a glyph in the hieroglyphic alphabet of the ancient Egyptians. Bauval explains that it would be impossible to know the true meaning of the symbol if one did not live the experience of the wagtail. He suggested:

> The full knowledge of the appearance of the wagtail in Egypt should evoke the idea and the moods of the autumn equinox, the receding waters of the Nile, the rich soil of the valley, the purity of the western deserts. (p. 51)

Here again is a demonstration of the material manifest reality more deeply sensed than from only its objective measurement. The ancient Egyptian language, as represented graphically by hieroglyphs, comprises not only phonetics but also a deep symbolism and representation of things more "unseen." Again, this manner of experiencing things was evident in the art of ancient Egypt as well as in their science.

The second author that began to open doors for me in my pursuit for a deeper understanding of the Egyptian psyche and cosmology was Jeremy Naydler. Similar to Bauval's insights, Naydler (1996) postulates that the ancient Egyptians believed that

> the physical universe had a "vertical dimension"; it reached up into, and included within itself, spiritual realities that for the modern consciousness are no longer a living experience. But for the ancient Egyptian, a metaphysical world poured into the physical, saturating it with meaning. (p. 11)

Looking at the remarkable scientific feats of the Egyptians through the lens that Bauval and Naydler present in these and others of their texts brought a completely different perspective of Egypt into my awareness.

Among other scholars whose works are referenced in this book is R. A. Schwaller de Lubicz (1998). His extensive study of the temple at Karnak resulted in his most impressive work, the massive two-volume *The Temple of Man: Apet of the South at Luxor*. Also cited are Graham Hancock and Bauval's (1996) *The Message of the Sphinx: A Quest for the Hidden Legacy of Mankind*; Edward Malkowski's (2007) research on Egyptian technology, specifically *The Spiritual Technology of Ancient Egypt: Sacred Science and the Mystery of Consciousness*; the aforementioned Christopher Dunn's (1998) seminal work *The Giza Power Plant: Technologies of Ancient Egypt*; and John Anthony West's (1993) interesting discoveries regarding the age of the Great Sphinx in relation to water erosion patterns.

Although there is much to be gleaned about ancient Egypt's people, Pharaohs' reigns, and customs from the more historical accounts published by the noted conventional Egyptologists of our time, the point of view of this book leans more toward the esoteric, as few modern conventional scholars give or gave *serious* attention to the magic, spirituality and the sacred science of Egypt—as Lewis Spence (1990) puts it, "Most of what has been written by Egyptologists on the subject of Egyptian magic has been penned on the assumption that magic is either a degraded form of religion, or its foundation" (p. 252).

There is, however, much pertinent material in older scholarly texts and articles written and published during a time (late 19th and early 20th centuries) when the line between dogmatic science and spiritual metaphysics was rather blurred. Even the great older Egyptologists such as E. A. Wallis Budge and Gaston Maspero, among a few others of equal stature, gave more credence to the subjective elements found in their topics of discussion and within their experience than modern Egyptologists; although, from my personal observation, a Victorian snobbishness is often present in many of these writings as well as an occasional obvious resistance to portray ideas that would be morally abhorrent to the Victorian European sensibility. The suppression of risqué ideas such as the fertility rituals of the Pharaoh that were practiced every evening in order to assure the return of the sun the following morning is reminiscent of Sigmund Freud's observation regarding the prevalence of neurosis in his Victorian practice due to the suppression of natural sexual drives. All things considered, the Victorian Egyptologists' writings and observations still contain wisps of the romantic notion of the mysteries of Egyptian culture and practice, thus preserving a bit of soul in the discourse. In other words, they don't typically dismiss ideas, theories, and concepts simply because modern reductionist science would find no place for them.

The development of this field of exploration and research was, however, an extremely slow process, and even as late as the early 20th century, it was difficult to distinguish serious Egyptologists from the tomb robbers of antiquity. The one thing that many of the Egyptologists, if not most, had in common was that they were Westerners, primarily European, and most, with the exceptions noted above, with scant regard for the subjective, spiritual, and metaphysical aspects of the ancient culture they called their passion. Once serious study began, ancient Egypt was largely examined through the lens of objectivist and reductionist science, which was predominantly European. Even today, Egyptology is largely viewed as a history of military campaigns, engineering feats, and other scientific accomplishments as well as superstitious ritual. Little attention was given to what many believe to be the primary thrust of the Egyptian psyche: determining humankind's position in the universe and how humans become gods themselves.

An ineffable quality inheres in the ancient Egyptians' view of existence, life, death, earthly activity, the universe, and the cosmos. Their myths and rituals can be translated, recited, and understood as narrative stories and processes, but their true meaning for the ancient Egyptians does not seem to be easily comprehended by the modern, materialist mind. Also, relatively recent discoveries (early 20th century) such as those documented in the controversial research of R. A. Schwaller de Lubicz (1961/1988, 1957/1998; Schwaller de Lubicz & Lamy, 1949/1977) have brought attention to a precision in temple construction, sculpture, geometry, and art that shows an almost obsessive consideration of detail beyond the needs of pragmatism and artistic freedom. Both the apparent depth of the ancient Egyptians' cosmology and their attention to such precision in their art, architecture, and engineering suggest a mystery of intention and meaning that belies conventional thought (Schwaller de Lubicz, 1961/1988).

We have only the manifest evidence of physical accomplishments that the ancient Egyptians created. It is unfortunate to realize that we know little about the manner in which they actually lived, loved, thought, and pondered—or what truly mattered to them philosophically and psychologically. Although their written history is quite complete in many ways, huge portions of it are missing from the existing records, and we come to conclusions without knowing a great many details about the way they lived and thought. We can only interpret the available evidence and speculate on the subjective lives of the Egyptians, and although there are extant examples of their poetry, stories, dreams, and even grocery and to-do lists, it is difficult not to compare their human, everyday life with other, more current, everyday lives with which we are familiar. To find similarities between an ancient way of life and a modern way of life would seemingly be an acceptable way of filling in the gaps where we have no evidence that convinces us of any differences. However, the design and construction of a large number of artifacts that the ancient Egyptians created belie our current understanding of the way the universe functions. It is then very difficult to settle on a conclusion that assumes the ancient Egyptians' way of life, in many respects, was similar to the way of life of other later cultures including our own. From the prolific evidence of unexplainable material objects, it seems the Egyptians had a way of thinking and subsequent execution of their ideas that defies anything we have come to understand. If this is true, then mainstream Egyptology may have largely missed the point regarding the basic nature of this culture and its impact on our current times.

This book posits that a third, equally important, crucial fundamental element is present in the cosmology of the ancient Egyptians that is equally responsible for the incredible feats materially presented by these people as well as the formidable wealth of spiritual insight they have brought to the rest of civilization. The first factor to be considered is the mind that conceived the thoughts, intentions, and ideas that created the mechanism for execution of these feats. This mechanism was then put into material action by the second crucial element—the body. The body takes action on matter in the material world and brings to physical manifestation the ideas and intentions the mind creates. The third element is the spirit, and in this context, I also venture to use the word *soul* as synonymous with *spirit*. This soul/spirit cannot be defined only by a belief or by a faith in an unknown, unseen force but must include spirit as an active and powerful, true and real force—no less in its nature and function than a material power. Modern Egyptology has essentially ignored this key element, and if given any sort of attention at all, it has been labeled as religion, magic, and superstition, and, with those labels, carries the limitations of their definitions.

Ancient Egyptians had no real use for what, in our current worldview, we call *religion*. They did not practice a religion as a separate set of beliefs, faiths, or rituals running alongside their everyday, secular, life. The ancient Egyptians were, in essence, their religion, and their religion was them. There was no separation, nothing set aside to believe, nothing to have faith in but the truth of their existence. Their world was not a dualistic world. It was a singular world, both inner and outer; just as we define today's duality, it was a singularity. There was a clear sacredness to all that the ancient Egyptians accomplished. In modern culture, *sacredness* is typically limited to religious or spiritual acts and experiences or possibly acts of a more artistic nature. Sacredness is considered as something inward and housed largely within one's personal psychology. In modern science, however, there is no proper place for sacredness, because it is not considered objective or material and cannot be reduced to its basic fundamental components. To the ancient Egyptians, sacredness comprised an inner knowingness—an innate consciousness of absolute Truth, natural and in harmony with their outer material world.

According to Schwaller de Lubicz (1961/1988, 1957/1998; Schwaller de Lubicz & Lamy, 1949/1977) and many other contemporary scholars (Bauval, 1999, 2008; Bauval & Brophy, 2011; Bauval & Gilbert, 1994; Dunn, 1998; Malkowski, 2007; Naydler, 1996, 2005; Schoch, 1999; Schoch & McNally, 2005; West, 1993), the Egyptians did not extract and discard a sacred quality from their science. This is the one single characteristic that clearly differentiates them from current culture. Obviously, differences are found between the unique customs, cosmologies, and art of each culture, but mainstream Egyptologists still insist that the ancient Egyptians were merely a primitive culture practicing superstitious beliefs much in the same manner that all unenlightened civilizations have done, and that everything else they did can fit neatly in what all humans have done or currently do, albeit considering the obvious uniqueness of being Egyptian and living in a time many centuries ago. "Surprisingly, however different the context and specifics might have been, work and play in Egypt's ancient culture closely resembled that of modern societies—at least until the nineteenth century, when machines took over the world" (Brier & Hobbs, 1999, p. 83). According to this conventional perspective, the incredible feats we see that the ancient Egyptians accomplished were executed within the laws of material science and Newtonian physics.

Evidence is mounting that shows the ancient Egyptians to be quite different from how we have perceived them to be. As mentioned previously, religion may not have been a religion to them at all or even a form of spirituality; it was simply a way of being. We have a much easier time relating to the ancient Egyptians through their quests for power, desire to acquire neighboring lands' riches, love of romance, art, faith in their beliefs about the cosmos and their gods, and other such familiar human drives and desires. It is far more difficult for us to grasp an understanding of a culture whose entire existence may have been seated in spirituality. Schwaller de Lubicz (1961/1988) said, "According to the evidence inscribed during a period of over four thousand years, ancient Egypt did not have a 'religion' as such; *it was religion in its entirety*, in the broadest and purest acceptation of the term" (p. 6). The intention behind all of their pursuits may not have been as we typically perceive the usual intention behind characteristic human endeavor. Sacredness was inherent in all that they did, and, most foreign to us in our modern materialist culture, there was sacredness to their science.

Ancient Egyptian sacred science—the harmony of the inner and outer world—would quite possibly answer the question of how the ancient Egyptians managed to manifest such incredible physical artifacts in art and architecture. The ancient Egyptians' world was infused with spirit; it was all living, all dynamic, and their inner, imaginal world danced effortlessly with the physical, material world. As portrayed by Naydler (1996), the psyches of the ancient Egyptians, both personally and collectively, were one and the same with the material world of matter they perceived outside of their physical bodies. This idea raises the question: What is psyche, and what is matter?

The psyche-to-matter problem has interested depth psychologists since Carl G. Jung (1952/1973) began theorizing about synchronicity in 1928 (Tarnas, 2006, p. 50), and indeed, the interest in this problem continues today with seemingly no less fervor than in Jung's time. Joseph Cambray (2009), an eminent Jungian analyst as well as a respected scholar, has written extensively on synchronicity and emergent property theory. Other modern scholars such as F. David Peat (1987), Victor Mansfield (1995), Ken Wilber (2001), and Stephen Braude (2007) have tackled the problem of psyche and matter with renewed vigor, not to mention the plethora of spiritual writers who also have a keen interest in the subject and, through a more metaphysical lens, explore the manner in which psyche possibly manipulates matter (e.g., Friedman, 1994; Goswami, Reed, & Goswami, 1993; Tart, 2009). Jungian theorist Marie-Louise von Franz (1992), in her book *Psyche and Matter*, wrote, "In the science of physics, the psyche mirrors matter, but that leads to the question: Can matter mirror the psyche?" (p. 18).

As can be imagined, this question has most likely been carefully scrutinized for quite some time. Researchers and scholars have found it in ancient texts such as the *Corpus Hermeticum*, attributed to a hypothetical historical figure, Hermes Trismegistus (Copenhaver, 1992), as well as in noncanonized Christian texts such as *The Gospel According to Mary Magdalene* (Doucet, 1990). The historical alchemical texts of Europe, Asia, and Egypt refer to transforming matter through chemical as well as psychical manipulation (Cavalli, 2010; von Franz, 1980; Linden, 2003; Maxwell-Stuart, 2008; Pregadio, 2006). The dozens of other resources related to the psyche-to-matter problem are too numerous to mention here, but this issue is discussed in more detail in Chapter 4.

Modern science describes the material world, and thus what we in modern times consider reality, as being made up only of physical particles and the energies associated with them. Ancient Egyptian sacred science suggests that physical reality is in fact infused with spirits and spirit (soul) and forces of the unseen, thus forming a wholly integrated reality, which includes the physical forms of nature as well as the unseen images, gods, goddesses, powers, symbols, and meanings that go beyond a rational, intelligent comprehension but present a harmonized inner and outer perception of reality.

Whereas the Egyptians did not have a dualistic cosmology that perceived their inner world as separate from and lesser than the outer world, our modern materialist way of thinking presumes there to be a distinct difference between the unseen (a realm beyond material existence) and the material world we call reality. Materializing an idea becomes a process of bringing a subjective thought into manifestation. There is, of course, nothing particularly novel about the concept of the transition from a thought idea to a physical manifestation; however, it is unusual how effectively the ancient Egyptians executed their physical creations and often, at times, in an unexplainable (through a physical explanation) manner. Although the creation of material representations of internal mental equivalents is not considered by scholars to be the extent of the Egyptian cosmology, it was deemed an important part of it. Testament to this assumption of importance is the magnificence of the extant monuments that are presently basking in the desert sun.

A greater knowledge of this Egyptian way of being could possibly open the door to a more efficacious form of psychotherapy—not merely to bring internal thoughts and images into form but also for better navigation through the reality of formal existence within the relationships we have with the material world in which we live. I am not merely suggesting an improvement in therapists' awareness of things internal, symbolic, or archetypal. Depth psychotherapy techniques as practiced today already adhere to these particular tenets. Suggested here is a more direct use of the concepts behind the ancient Egyptian way of interfacing with the world, both external and internal. This heightened connection of both the therapist and the patient with the inner imaginal world would result in a transformation of the outer world, which becomes imbued with symbolic content of inner values, truths, and intentions—all in line with the Egyptian concept of *ma'at*. Simply defined, *ma'at* is order out of chaos—a cosmic intention that is, at its core, benevolent, just, and divine (Naydler, 1996, pp. 94–97). In the outer world, or the world of form and material substance, Egyptians spent their entire lives working toward *ma'at*. In his book *Temple of the Cosmos: The Ancient Egyptian Experience of the Sacred*, Jeremy Naydler said, "Ancient Egyptians were constantly exhorted to 'do *ma'at*' and to 'speak *ma'at*.' By so doing, they came closer to the divine, kingly principle in themselves, and thus transcended the merely human and contingent" (p. 96).

This proposition is not meant to suggest a dogmatic view consisting of judgmental values or truths but simply a methodology following the inner *nous* or sacred knowingness that will result in a greater balance and alignment with harmony and evolutionary growth. At the very least, reflecting on the concepts behind the ancient Egyptians' way of engaging with their world could provide a deeper understanding and integration of the reality of existence that holds the inner world just as worthy of consideration as the outer.

References

Bauval, R. (1999). *Secret chamber: The quest for the hall of records*. London, England: Century.

Bauval, R. (2008). *The Egypt code*. New York, NY: Disinformation.

Bauval, R., & Brophy, T. G. (2011). *Black genesis: The prehistoric origins of ancient Egypt*. Rochester, VT: Bear.

Bauval, R., & Gilbert, A. (1994). *The Orion mystery: Unlocking the secrets of the pyramids*. New York, NY: Crown.

Braude, S. E. (2007). *The gold leaf lady and other parapsychological investigations*. Chicago, IL: University of Chicago Press.

Brier, B., & Hobbs, A. H. (1999). *Daily life of the ancient Egyptians*. Westport, CT: Greenwood Press.

Cambray, J. (2009). *Synchronicity: Nature and psyche in an interconnected universe*. College Station, TX: Texas A & M University Press.

Cavalli, T. F. (2010). *Embodying Osiris: The secrets of alchemical integration*. Wheaton, IL: Theosophical.

Copenhaver, B. P. (Trans. & Ed.). (1992). *Hermetica: The Greek* Corpus hermeticum *and the Latin* Asclepius *in a new English translation, with notes and introduction*. Cambridge, England: Cambridge University Press.

Doucet, C. (1990). *The gospel according to Mary Magdalene*. Windsor, ON: Black Moss Press.

Dunn, C. (1998). *The Giza power plant: Technologies of ancient Egypt*. Santa Fe, NM: Bear.

Friedman, N. (1994) *Bridging science and spirit: Common elements in David Bohm's physics, the perennial philosophy and Seth*. St. Louis, MO: Moment Point Press.

Goswami, A., Reed, R. E., & Goswami, M. (1993). *The self-aware universe: How consciousness creates the material world*. New York, NY: Putnam.

Hancock, G., & Bauval, R. (1996). *The message of the Sphinx: A quest for the hidden legacy of mankind*. New York, NY: Crown.

Jung, C. G. (1973). Synchronicity: An acausal connecting principle. In H. Read, M. Fordham, & G. Adler (Eds.), *The collected works of C. G. Jung* (R. F. C. Hull, Trans.) (Vol. 8, pp. 417–531). Princeton, NJ: Princeton University Press. (Original work published 1952)

Linden, S. J. (2003). *The alchemy reader: From Hermes Trismegistus to Isaac Newton*. Cambridge, UK: Cambridge University Press.

Malkowski, E. F. (2007). *The spiritual technology of ancient Egypt: Sacred science and the mystery of consciousness*. Rochester, VT: Inner Traditions.

Mansfield, V. (1995). *Synchronicity, science, and soul-making: Understanding Jungian synchronicity through physics, Buddhism, and philosophy*. Chicago, IL: Open Court.

Maxwell-Stuart, P. G. (2008). *The chemical choir*. London, England: Continuum.

Naydler, J. (1996). *Temple of the cosmos: The ancient Egyptian experience of the sacred*. Rochester, VT: Inner Traditions.

Naydler, J. (2005). *Shamanic wisdom in the pyramid texts: The mystical tradition of ancient Egypt.* Rochester, VT: Inner Traditions.

Peat, F. D. (1987). *Synchronicity: The bridge between matter and mind.* New York, NY: Bantam Books.

Pregadio, F. (2006). *Great clarity: Daoism and alchemy in early medieval China.* Stanford, CA: Stanford University Press.

Schoch, R. M. (with McNally, R. A.). (1999). *Voices of the rocks: A scientist looks at catastrophes and ancient civilizations.* New York, NY: Harmony Books.

Schoch, R. M., & McNally, R. A. (2005). *Pyramid quest: Secrets of the Great Pyramid and the dawn of civilization.* New York, NY: Tarcher/Penguin.

Schwaller de Lubicz, R. A. (1988). *Sacred science: The king of pharaonic theocracy* (A. VandenBroeck & G. VandenBroeck, Trans.). Rochester, VT: Inner Traditions International. (Original work published 1961)

Schwaller de Lubicz, R. A. (1998). *The temple of man: Apet of the South at Luxor* (2 vols.) (R. Lawlor & D. Lawlor, Trans.). Rochester, VT: Inner Traditions. (Original work published 1957)

Schwaller de Lubicz, R. A., & Lamy, L. (1977). *The temple in man: The secrets of ancient Egypt* (R. Lawlor & D. Lawlor, Trans.). New York, NY: Autumn Press. (Original work published 1949)

Spence, L. (1990). *Ancient Egyptian myths and legends.* New York: Dover Publications.

Tarnas, R. (2006). *Cosmos and psyche: Intimations of a new world view.* New York, NY: Viking.

Tart, C. T. (2009). *The end of materialism: How evidence of the paranormal is bringing science and spirit together.* Oakland, CA: Noetic Books/New Harbinger.

von Franz, M.-L. (1980). *Alchemy: An introduction to the symbolism and the psychology.* Toronto, Canada: Inner City Books.

von Franz, M.-L. (1992). *Psyche and matter.* Boston, MA: Shambhala.

West, J. A. (1993). *Serpent in the sky: The high wisdom of ancient Egypt.* Wheaton, IL: Quest Books.

Wilber, K. (Ed.). (2001). *Quantum questions: Mystical writings of the world's great physicists.* Boston, MA: Shambhala.

2

THE MIRACLES OF ANCIENT EGYPT

In the blistering heat of the summer of 1798, Napoleon Bonaparte invaded Egypt by sea via the coastal city of Alexandria. Although the strategy to acquire Egypt as a French colony was rationalized on several fronts—particularly with the intention of weakening Great Britain's Asian trade capabilities—Napoleon also had a less militaristic obsession with the mysterious region. Along with the 40,000 men he carried to the Egyptian delta on board his hundreds of ships, Napoleon hosted an entourage of notable men of science, art, archeology, and engineering. His goal was to document as much as he could of Egypt's ancient history, geology, flora, and fauna and, with this robust and rigorous scientific investigation, bring the spirit of European Enlightenment to the region.

Although entering a country a mere 2,000 miles from their French homeland, Napoleon and his men were crossing a threshold into a region possibly as strange to them as a distant planet. Invading foreign lands was nothing new to Napoleon and his troops, but the drive to conquer the home of the pyramids held a special place in the psyche of the French general. Napoleon apparently was fascinated with the history of ancient Egypt and took a special interest in the work of his scientific contingent. Even though the European Enlightenment was proclaimed as a movement away from superstition and an embracing of scientific order and rationality, Napoleon himself seems to have been obsessed with the magic and metaphysical perspectives of this alluring land he now occupied.

More than likely an apocryphal story, legend has it that Napoleon spent several hours in the King's Chamber of Khufu's Great Pyramid, and, upon entering the chamber, had asked to be left alone. When he finally did exit the smooth, granite-paneled walls of the alleged burial room, he was quite shaken and refused to speak of his experience. He went further in his attempt to erase the event from the curious minds of those who accompanied him by requesting that no one ever speak of it to him again. According to the legend, while he was on his deathbed, his command of silence was broken, and a close friend asked him to recount the tale. Napoleon began to speak but ultimately hesitated and then fell silent after mumbling to his friend, "There is no point in telling, you would not believe me" ("Napoleon's Visit," 2014; "Napoleon and the Great Pyramid," 2014). Though this is a curious and intriguing story, its truth or fallacy does not alter Napoleon's importance in the resurrection of Egypt from the sands of time back into the global consciousness as a viable and worthy subject of study and reflective contemplation.

Although Europeans, including the French, had had scant presence in Egypt for centuries, Napoleon's experience in this enchanted land presents one important perspective of the modern (post-18th-century) Western fascination with the magic and mystery of Egypt. Napoleon's conquest and occupation of this part of the world, which lasted only three years, ushered in a new view of the ancient Egyptian mystique. He was the first prominent European to bring the objective powers of observation of the European Enlightenment to the world of the pharaohs; moreover, his exploration led to the milestone discovery of the Rosetta Stone, which, at the least, began to crack an opening into the previously untouchable quality of an ancient civilization's undecipherable language.

During Napoleon's expedition, one of his soldiers discovered a granodiorite stele near the town of Rashid (Western name, Rosetta), where early Christians had moved it from its original temple site. The stone was immediately considered unique, with its etched inscription of three distinct languages, one of them Greek. Twenty years passed, however, before all three passages were translated, including a hieroglyphic version of the Greek text, by Jean-François Champollion in Paris in 1822. Probably no other single event in the history of Egyptology has had the impact of this translation. Suddenly, after thousands of years of silence, the Egyptian hieroglyph system of writing had an explicable voice. With this newfound ability to understand the thousands of hieroglyphic inscriptions in artwork and on the walls of ancient Egyptian temples, mastabas, and monuments, a documented history of Egypt's kings and queens, military campaigns, funerary practices, religion, and art started to take form. Egyptology began to develop as a scientific discipline as the burgeoning field of archeology shifted from a band of looters and collectors of treasure for a monetary return to a serious group of scientists interested in history, culture, and anthropology. Napoleon's expedition was the first incidence of Western culture seriously penetrating the mysterious land since Alexander the Great and the Ptolemaic Greek period followed by the Roman conquest, which essentially ended Pharaonic rule of the region in approximately 30 BCE.

The exceptional results of Napoleon's campaign into Egypt were presented in the brilliant *Description de l'Egypte* (Napoleon I, Jomard, Lelorgne de Savigny, & Fourier, 1809–1829), originally published in 23 volumes starting in the year 1809, with the final volume appearing in 1829. This concerted effort of over 2,000 scientists and artists was, at the time of its publication and release to the public, the most comprehensive documentation of Egypt known to the world.

This Herculean investigation by Napoleon's contingent into Egypt presents an important and soulful expression of the Western mind and heart as it interfaced with the manifest realities as well as the mysteries of the ancient Egyptian world.

Napoleon departed Egypt in 1799, leaving the country in quite a political mess. The French occupied Egypt for only a few more years (the British took control in 1801, but their rule also lasted only a few years). The modern discipline of Egyptology, as a science, began to take form in the first few decades of the 19th century. Napoleon's contribution, with the publication of the *Description de l'Egypte* between 1809 and 1829, brought the mysteries of the region to the hearts and minds of Europe in a way that had not previously been realized. As mentioned before, the deciphering of the Rosetta Stone (in the 1820s) also allowed for a more serious European engagement in Egyptology as an academic pursuit.

Before any sort of earnest study of Egypt's monuments and artifacts took place, several quite colorful characters invaded the country for the adventure and sport of treasure hunting, excavation, and the intrigue of archeological discovery. One such figure was "The Great Belzoni"—Giovanni Battista Belzoni (1778–1823). Belzoni, born in Padua, Italy, was a hulk of a man known for his formidable height (6' 7") and circus-man strength—Belzoni actually worked in the circus as a strongman, with his wife, purported to be a strongwoman, during the early 1800s. Belzoni claimed to have been trained during schooling years in hydraulic engineering and was first drawn to Egypt through a desire to present to Muhammad Ali, then pasha of Egypt (1815), a water pump system he had devised to raise the waters of the Nile. The system seemed to have been a success, but the pasha passed on its utilization. Belzoni was then stuck in Egypt with little to occupy his time until, through the influences of the orientalist J. L. Burckhardt, he was sent by the Egyptian British consul, Henry Salt, to the Ramesseum at Thebes. Here he accomplished one of the tasks for which he is most famous—the removal of a 9-ton bust of Ramesses II and its subsequent shipping to the British Museum.

The Great Belzoni went on to perform other Herculean feats, such as the removal of tons of sand from the entrance to the Abu Simbel complex, excavations at Karnak, and opening the crypt at the burial site of Seti I (still often referred to as "Belzoni's Tomb"), He was given credit for being the first modern man to gain access to the second pyramid of Giza, Khafre's pyramid, and to explore its chambers. He also participated in expeditions to the Red Sea as well as into the desert oasis of Bahariya. "Bull in a China shop" could be a quite fitting description of Belzoni, as his archeological methods were anything but delicate. His whole intent seems to have been to pry out of the Egyptian rock and sand anything he could, using any method he had at his disposal. He created a rather terrible reputation for himself among other explorers and officials of the time, predominantly French and Italian, due to his reckless methods that often destroyed more than they preserved. However, the delicate art of archeology was in its infancy at the time, and there were few in Belzoni's company who conducted themselves much differently.

Another somewhat illustrious explorer of Egypt was James Burton (1788–1862). Born in London, Burton was educated at Trinity College, Cambridge and worked for the architect Sir John Soane from 1815 to 1822. During this period he met up with the Egyptologists Sir John Gardner Wilkinson, Edward William Lane, and Sir William Gell and subsequently was invited by Pasha Mohammad Ali to come to Egypt as a mineralogist (although he had no experience or training as such) and to participate in the Geological Survey of Egypt, primarily to prospect for coal. Much like Belzoni, Burton eventually was led to other pursuits and began a rather mysterious and adventurous tour of Egypt and her ancient sites. From 1825 to 1834, Burton seemed to disappear, and little is known of his activities, other than his wanderings through the deserts of Egypt. Between 1825 and 1828, he did manage to complete the publication of a volume of hieroglyphic inscriptions, *Excerpta Hieroglyphica*, but was out of touch with the European world until he showed up in England, on December 25, 1835, with a collection of exotic animals (including a giraffe), servants, and slaves. He also brought home a wife, Andreana, who was a Greek slave whom he had purchased sometime during his travels in Egypt. His subsequent marriage to Andreana caused his somewhat snobbish Victorian family to disown him. As a result of this ostracism, he accumulated quite a bit of debt and was forced to sell all of his Egyptian antiquities and books. He held onto a mummy and a coffin, which is still on display at Liverpool's World Museum.

Burton's contribution to Egyptology is varied and substantial. He traveled through much of Egypt along the Nile River, from Cairo to Abu Simbel, working at the Mortuary Temple of Ramesses II, the Mortuary Temple of Ramesses III, the Temple of Amun-Ra, and the Temple of Amenophis III. He also excavated a number of tombs in the Valley of the Kings necropolis, and he is credited as being the first explorer in modern times to have entered the now-famous KV 5 tomb. At the time of Burton's entrance into the tomb, it was found to be quite small; however, over a century later, in 1995, Egyptologist Kent Weeks excavated past Burton's initial venture to expose what is now considered to be the largest tomb in the valley and the most important find since the discovery of the Tomb of Tutankhamen in 1922 by Howard Carter. Burton also did quite a bit of excavation at Kom Ombo, Aswan, Philae, Medina Habu, and Karnak.

One of the first Egyptologists to have a notably more acceptable method of research, discovery, and excavation was German Egyptologist Karl Richard Lepsius (1810–1884). Lepsius began his study of the pyramids at Giza and the surrounding areas utilizing methods of precise documentation with academic acumen. He studied Greek and Roman archeology at the University of Leipzig as well as attending lectures by Jean Letronne, who was an early disciple of Jean-François Champollion of Rosetta Stone fame. Lepsius scoured Europe for anything Egyptian and regularly attended Egyptian museum exhibits and presentations as well as lectures and other academic Egyptian conferences. His avid interest drove him at a time when an education in Egyptology had to be eked out in ways other than through formal education in Europe's graduate university programs. Armed with this extensive self-taught knowledge of Egypt and his hard-earned expertise in the translation of ancient Egyptian hieroglyphs, Lepsius headed out to Egypt in 1842 with the blessing of Friedrich Wilhelm IV of Prussia, who had commissioned him to bring back to Germany a thorough understanding and documentation of the mysteries of Egypt, in addition to as much of her material riches he could lay his hands on.

Lepsius was the first, since Napoleon's entourage swept through the lands of Egypt 40 years earlier, to bring such scholarly and detailed attention to the region. Lepsius brought with him an English architect, James Wild, and the artist Joseph Bonomi as well as others of various disciplines to record the monuments he encountered and to procure museum booty to cart back to his homeland. Lepsius spent the months following his arrival in 1842 exploring Abusir, Saqqara, Dahshur, and Giza, primarily engaged in the discovery and study of the pyramid structures found at those sites. He is credited for the discovery of about sixty-seven pyramids as well as numerous tombs of the aristocracy of ancient Egypt. Although several notable scholars and explorers had come before him, such as Richard H. Vyse and John S. Perring as well as the Franco-Tuscan expedition of 1828 led by Jean-François Champollion himself, Lepsius is recognized by modern scholars as being the first to study the pyramids in such depth and with such academic meticulousness.

Auguste Mariette, a Frenchman who lived most of his life in Egypt and died there in 1881, was one of the first Egyptologists to fall so deeply in love with the country of his passions that he devoted most of his life to learning what he could about its ancient past, customs, and monuments. Mariette was born at Boulogne-sur-Mer in 1821. His cousin, Nestor L'Hôte, who travelled with Champollion to Egypt during the Franco-Tuscan expedition of 1828, died in 1842 leaving his papers and drawings to be filed and sorted by Auguste. As Auguste worked through this mountain of sketches, he began to develop a deep passion for Egypt and decided to devote his life to Egyptology. Like Lepsius, an autodidact, Mariette devoted his time to the study of hieroglyphics and Coptic, an ancient Egyptian language of the later period.

In 1850, the 29-year-old Mariette headed to Egypt by the request of the French government to search for and acquire ancient manuscripts of Coptic, Syriac, Arabic, and Ethiopian origin for the Louvre museum. The Louvre was concerned about keeping its current supremacy over other collections and wished to sponsor a serious effort to acquire more material for its coffers. When Mariette arrived in the arid and profoundly alien landscape of Egypt, he did little better than to become a complete failure. Mostly due to his inexperience in the fast-paced and vicious antiquities market, Mariette was faced with the dismal prospect of returning home empty handed. He instead set out into the desert to satisfy his thirst for Egypt, befriended a Bedouin tribe who knew the desert, and stumbled across what seemed to him to be an ideal spot to begin an excavation. Upon noticing a lone sphinx statue with its head thrust above the desert sand, he gathered a cadre of Egyptian workers and began to dig. Thus, about a year after landing in Egypt, Mariette made a vital archeological discovery—the celebrated avenue of the sphinxes, and a little later, the discovery of the Serapeum at Saqqara, the Apis bull burial site described in Chapter 1.

Several years after these initial discoveries, political intrigue ensued as Mariette was accused of theft and destruction of sacred sites by competitive diggers and the government of Egypt. He decided to rebury many of his finds to keep his competitors from illegally seizing his discoveries. After eluding the scroungers, he would re-excavate his original dig and recover what he had previously discovered. Over the next four years, Mariette sent home to the Louvre not the manuscripts they had originally sent him to Egypt to procure but, instead, many far more precious artifacts of ancient Egypt. Mariette was known for working with the local authorities, and he and the French government struck up a deal whereby the Louvre received 50% of his finds, and the Egyptian government received the other 50%. Upon his return to France, Mariette brought with him 230 crates of goods, and an equal amount remained in Egypt.

Mariette did not dally for long in France: within a year, he was back in Egypt on the resolve of the Egyptian government who offered him, in 1858, the position of conservator of Egyptian monuments. Mariette continued his career in Egypt with dizzying success and accomplishment. Never before had Egypt seen so much concentrated effort to turn Egyptology from a pseudo-science filled with glory seekers, thieves, and museum-subsidized adventurers into a respectable, organized, and ethically minded discipline made up of scientists, researchers, and academicians. Things were far from perfect, but Mariette did usher in a new ideal of Egyptology.

Gaston Maspero (1846–1916), a fellow Frenchman, came to Egypt in 1880—a bit later in life than his predecessor Auguste Mariette, whom he met in Paris a decade or so before his relocation to Egypt. A few months after his arrival, upon Mariette's death, Maspero succeeded him as director-general of excavations and antiquities. Maspero was predominantly an academic linguist holding several posts as professor at various educational institutions. He was also instrumental, in his government post, in the curtailment of runaway looting and the illegal export of antiquities by tourists and collectors—many of whom were actually working for European and American museums. Being the diplomat that he was, Maspero was skilled at working with museum directors and others, allowing certain exports and condemning others. He was considered to be pragmatic and fair and created a reasonable process working within the limitations presented to him.

Maspero is probably better known as an administrator and politician within the bureaucracy of the Egyptian government than as a field archeologist. He established an international awareness for the collection and exhibition of Egyptian antiquities through an organized and efficient system of supplying museums with the artifacts they most desired, while encouraging the Egyptians to take pride in their heritage and build up their own local collections. Maspero was also a prolific writer and produced a number of books and pamphlets.

E. A. Wallis Budge (1857–1934) was a zealous writer as well, who produced many authoritative volumes on the ancient Egyptians' religion and art and their particular way of life. Budge was an Englishman who never held a government post in the French-dominated Egyptology contingent. He was, however, an inexhaustible collector of goods for the British Museum, where he held several posts during his lifetime. Budge is reputed to have supplied the bulk of the British Museum's holdings in artifacts of the Ancient Near East collections, having picked up anything that he could during his numerous trips to Egypt. Budge is probably best known by contemporary alternative Egypt aficionados as the man who translated the seminal *Egyptian Book of the Dead* (1899b). This was a project close to the heart of the man who claimed to have believed in ghosts and the spirit world. Many colleagues and contemporaries of Budge's who had lost their faith in Christianity became ardent followers of Budge's literary work on the occult, mystical religions, and the paranormal.

It is in these works of Budge's that we get a glimpse of the importance of Egyptian religion and spirituality. Budge and a handful of theosophist scholars were the first to pay attention to more than the materialist offerings of this profoundly intriguing culture. His research on Egypt's religious writings, tomb art, and magic provides the seeds of an ultimate understanding, or at least an informed awareness, of the Egyptian concept of sacred science.

Possibly the first person to take serious scientific interest in the engineering feats of the ancient Egyptians was William Matthew Flinders Petrie, the son of an engineer. He first traveled to Egypt in 1880 to survey the Giza plateau and later to head up excavations at various sites. Throughout his work in Egypt, he made exacting studies of the construction of the pyramids and other ancient sites, taking precise measurements of blocks, level deviations, cardinal placements, drilling of holes in granite and limestone, and the creation of engravings and bas-reliefs. Petrie concluded that the Egyptians must have used drills, saws, and lathes to produce the objects they built and the art and writing in stone they created. He observed details in construction such as drilling-bit striations, saw cuts, and various other effects from copper or bronze tools. Much evidence to support Petrie's findings has been discovered, including a piece of a copper saw blade safely tucked away in his museum in London.

Christopher Dunn, a modern-day engineer who has repeated some of Petrie's work in assessing engineering feats of the ancient Egyptians, claims that Petrie suggested the Egyptian's use of these tools were beyond their technological acumen and rivaled the technology of his own day (1880s). Dunn, who is not an Egyptologist or a trained research scientist, may be correct in his assertions, but it is impossible to know exactly what Petrie was thinking at the time. Thirty years after the 1883 publication of his *The Pyramids and Temples of Gizeh*, Petrie did recant some of his earlier claims in his book *The Arts and Crafts of Ancient Egypt* (1910), and suggested different methods of cutting, drilling, and shaping than what he had originally proposed.

Although more recent efforts have successfully emulated the Egyptians' supposed methods of cutting, sawing, and drilling, much controversy persists among alternative researchers regarding these speculated techniques. These skeptics consider some of the statuary to be much too precise in their execution to have been created by such crude methods. Petrie's first conjectures regarding diamond-tipped tools had to be abandoned due to the lack of any evidence whatsoever of diamonds or diamond dust in excavations. However, the results of some sort of method, whatever it may be, are clearly available to examine and ponder in their near-perfect precision and ineffable meticulousness in construction. Christopher Dunn, among others, insists that there had to have been some currently unknown technology available to the ancient Egyptians in order to create such exactitude in their art, statuary, and sarcophagi or such mammoth undertaking in the building of their larger monuments such as temples and pyramids.

This limited survey of Egyptology and its practitioners in the 19th and early 20th centuries ends here. Clearly, dozens of other prominent Egyptologists visited Egypt during this time and after (notably, the most famous of all Egyptologists, Howard Carter, who discovered the tomb of Tutankhamen in 1922), but the men surveyed here suffice to illustrate the point I am attempting to make about the foundation and roots of Western Egyptology. I end this survey with Petrie because I believe he was the first explorer who began to question the origins, methods, techniques, and abilities of the ancient culture that supposedly had created all that now sits in the Egyptian desert, using only the tools and knowledge that their limited status as a so-called primitive culture allowed them. Petrie's meticulous documentation and observation, with its penchant for detail that only an engineer can possess, presented to the world information about ancient Egypt and her artifacts that had not yet been fathomed. Whereas most before him focused their attention on the physical enormity of what they had discovered, Petrie also focused on the minutia, cataloguing thousands of variants in design, material, and methods of construction. Petrie was one of the first to take notice of the extreme precision and miniscule tolerances within which the Egyptians created their art, statuary, and monuments. He questioned the conventional views regarding the tools the Egyptians must have possessed in order to build with such sureness, and he painstakingly documented his observations. With Petrie, a new paradigm began to develop, and even though more than seventy-five years had to pass before these alternative views of ancient Egypt gained any sort of exposure to the general public, it was nonetheless a beginning.

As mentioned, this brief outline of the early history of Egyptology in Egypt illustrates the predominantly Christian European, patriarchal nature of the field at that time. Egyptology as we know it today has this Victorian sensibility as its foundation, initially only concerned with the monetary value of stolen antiquities possessed through a largely aggressive bravura steeped in a masculine paradigm of competition and expression of power. Little serious attention was given to the advanced spirituality of the ancient Egyptians, as most encounters with this element of the culture were met with derision and a Victorian–Christian distaste for primitive superstition and eroticism. Although these early explorers were quite taken by the beauty of the art, design, and architecture they encountered in their work, they were more impressed with the enormity of the physical effort required to create the hundreds of extant temples, monuments, and statuary they uncovered. Even today, serious academic study of ancient Egypt concerns itself more with the procession of Pharaonic dynasties, social customs, mummification, military campaigns, and temple construction than with cosmology, spirituality, Egyptian magic, and sacred science.

These men were, however, more emotionally affected by their work than most accounts give them credit. The writings of Budge, Maspero, Petrie, and others sometimes convey an almost misty-eyed romanticism. Their souls were gripped by something unseen in Egypt that went beyond museum acquisitions, government politics, and academic honors bestowed by their affiliate European universities. In Budge's *Egyptian Magic*, he described the early Egyptians' sense of the cosmos:

> Egyptian magic dates from the time when the predynastic and prehistoric dwellers in Egypt believed that the earth, and the underworld, and the air, and the sky were peopled with countless beings, visible and invisible, which were held to be friendly or unfriendly to man according as the operations of nature, which they were supposed to direct, were favourable or unfavourable to him. (1899a, p. viii)

Although an interest in heathen, non-Christian religious practice existed in Budge's time, these practices were most often considered seated in the backwaters of primitive superstition. Here, Budge's writing again presents interesting insight regarding the supposed superstitious nature of these early Egyptian beliefs as being primarily due to the culture's naïveté and innocence based on a limited and ultimately unscientific understanding.

However, a deeper meaning and purpose underlying the ancient Egyptians' mystical way of viewing their universe was essentially ignored by Budge—at least in his academic writing—as it was possibly considered to be unfounded and purposeless and was then cast aside as merely curious and quaint. Although Budge did possess a keen interest in things "unseen," he probably joined most other academics of the time in the rejection of the possibility that any true and meaningful purpose could be behind these paranormal anomalies. I believe it would have been difficult for him, or anyone else at the time who was engaged in the serious work of Egyptology, to believe that the ancient Egyptians' spiritual views and practices could have had any direct influence on their ability to create the unprecedented physical world they created.

Gaston Maspero also wrote several important books during his time in Egypt, but the work that is most relevant to the thesis presented here is his *Art in Egypt*, published in 1912. Maspero's scholarship again supports the idea, found even in these very early studies and academic assessments, that ancient Egypt's art is impossible to separate from its religion and that, in fact, all of Egyptian culture was religion. Writing about the decline of the Egyptian culture with the advent of European/Christian dominance, he asserted, "The art of Egypt, like its literature, its science, its current civilization, was one with its religion" (p. 301). Here, another seed was planted that would grow in support of later ideas regarding Egyptian sacred science, to be discussed in detail in subsequent chapters.

Several other scholars and authors of this period, mid- to late 19th century to the mid-20th centuries, presented, in addition to a view of the materialistic, dynastic elements of ancient Egypt, a more esoteric perspective. This period was rife with spiritual thinking and alternate paths to enlightenment. Many were breaking out of the dogmatic restrictions of traditional religions and investigating other ways to find God, meaning and purpose to life, and individual spirituality, thus creating an interest in the Egyptian concept of religion and reality. For example, Helena Petrovna Blavatsky (1831–1891), a significant figure in the world of esoteric studies and spirituality, initially believed that all esoteric knowledge emanated from ancient Egypt. She changed her view slightly later in her career to focus more on Tibet as the primary source of this knowledge, but always honored some significant roots in Egypt.

Blavatsky along with Colonel Henry Steel Olcott, William Quan Judge, and several others founded the Theosophical Society in New York City in 1875. This organization was devoted to the study of theosophy, a belief in the unity of all nature and reality, and was engaged in the search for the essence of divinity, profound philosophical realities, and the mysteries of the universe. Along with Blavatsky and Judge (1951), other respected scholars and researchers in the esoteric fields who contributed to the Theosophical Society's publication, *The Theosophical Path*, were Katherine Tingley (1992) and Charles J. Ryan (1911, 1939). In Ryan's (1911) article "The New Egyptology and the Theosophical Records," for example, he made clear that, even at this early stage of inquiry, the more esoteric thinkers were questioning the conventional conclusions about the age of the pyramids and the Egyptian culture itself. Ryan wrote:

> According to the Theosophical records the Great Pyramid was built long before the fifth millennium BC. There are many mysteries connected with that most stupendous work of man, which have not yet been suspected by the Egyptologists, not the least of which is the problem of its date and its builder. (p. 19)

Questions regarding the actual date of the construction of the pyramids and who may have actually built them are ultimately not a concern in this book; however, allowing for a theory that essentially is open to nonphysical causation is indeed relevant. If the pyramids were not constructed as burial temples and if they were not constructed using the conventional theory of monumental manpower, it seems prudent to consider other nonmaterial elements such as a method of manipulating matter through the psyche using energies that do not conform to the typical materialist's definition of reality. This theory, in fact, is a central theme of this book and presents the thesis that the mind, or psyche, of an individual has a direct influence on the physical universe he or she occupies.

The study of the ancient Egyptians continued on into the 20th century in much the same fashion as it started, but became more and more sophisticated, academic in nature, ethically disciplined, and accepted as a true science. At the same time, the perceptions of Egyptology became less and less mysterious, evocative, romantic, and spiritual. There were still many who found ancient Egypt's true gift to the world to be in her myths, her spirituality, and her view of the cosmos, but few in the academic and conventional science of Egyptology have seen past the primitive and superstitious nature of Egypt's obsessions with the afterlife, mummification, art, magic, and religion.

Relatively recently, however, some serious scientific study has been achieved by a handful of "out-of-the-box" thinkers, scientists, and mystics. Although they do not all see eye to eye, their work in the alternate history field has been substantial and influential for those interested in a worldview contrary to mainstream archeology. In the late 20th century and ongoing, the engineer Christopher Dunn, as mentioned earlier, has continued the work of Flinders Petrie through his own thorough, scientific investigation of the engineering prowess of the ancient Egyptians. Dunn has had the advantage of the use of more sophisticated measuring instruments and has determined, through his own collected evidence, that the engineering achievements demonstrated by the Egyptians are in some cases beyond today's technology. Dunn insisted that they had to have had at their disposal such sophisticated equipment as sonic drills, precision planning and lapping equipment, and large saw wheels that would rival, in their sophistication and efficacy, the tools that are available today. Dunn believes that the modern efforts to emulate ancient Egyptian engineering have utterly failed to reach the high standards of perfection the ancients accomplished. Dunn's work has been met with extreme derision by the orthodox Egyptology community, which discredits most of what he has to say.

In the desert sands of Abu Rawash, approximately 5 miles north of the Giza plateau, sitting in plain view is a large slab of rose granite, approximately 4 feet by 3 feet in surface dimension and 8 inches thick, cut smoothly on one side and showing obvious saw grooves on its surface. What makes this piece of granite unique, among the thousands of other pieces of cut granite found in this part of Egypt, are the mysterious markings etched into its surface. Dunn and other engineers he has consulted say that these markings—their width, depth, the distance between them, and the manner in which they were made—suggest the use of a very large cutting saw, a wheel approximately 35 feet in diameter (Dunn, 2008). Evidence of the existence of such a saw cannot be found, and, obviously, a saw such as this does not fit into the historical context. I visited Abu Rawash myself during my second trip to Egypt in 2009 and examined this mysterious granite slab, as described in more detail at the end of this chapter. Dozens of other mysteriously cut stones can be found in Egypt that may not indicate so clearly a questionable form of creation but, nonetheless, comprise qualities that are difficult to attribute to the mainstream conclusions regarding their construction.

Dunn's most famous as well as most controversial speculations address the use of the Great Pyramid on the Giza plateau. He rejects the idea that the pyramid was built as a tomb for the Early Kingdom Pharaoh Kufu, as do many alternative Egyptologists. He does, however, theorize the sensational, claiming that the pyramids were giant power-processing plants. Dunn's explanation of these mechanical systems, as found in his *The Giza Powerplant* (1998), is quite compelling, as he answers many questions that have confounded conventional Egyptology since the beginning of Egyptian study. (Needless to say, conventional Egyptology patently rejects his theory.) His ideas are not based on supernatural phenomena but, instead, are well-formulated, scientific mechanisms and processes that only an engineer such as Dunn would be able to conceptualize. He and others have even built small-scale models of his machine (certain aspects of it, at least) that do function as anticipated. His conjectures, considered by many to be reckless, do open up some serious questions—and, if true, answer other serious questions that have been baffling archeologists since the beginning of ancient Egyptian inquiry.

As noted, Dunn's views clearly fly in the face of conventional archeology and Egyptology. For years, conventional Egyptologists have had to battle what they claim to be the lack of scientific rigor in the presentation of these alternative histories and a complete disregard for context, which is a hallmark of robust archeological research. If Dunn's unusual theories do not fall within the boundaries of known science, they are then dismissed and not even seriously considered. Although there have been a few isolated and notable public debates over these theories, conventional Egyptologists have a tendency simply to ignore them. It seems that no importance is placed on rationally disputing an idea that is, by its very nature, considered irrational. John Anthony West (1993), in his book *Serpent in the Sky: The High Wisdom of Ancient Egypt*, had this to say:

> In Egyptology, as in so many modern disciplines, all questions are believed to have "rational" answers. If no evidence is available to provide a rational answer, the customary solution is to trivialize the mystery. In many academic circles triviality is a synonym for reason. (p. 13)

If Dunn is correct, or even partially correct, his theory places the ancient Egyptians in a category entirely out of context with prevailing Egyptology in particular, and the history and evolution of humankind in general.

While conducting the research for this book, I communicated with several conventional Egyptologists and asked them to comment on Dunn's work. A few of them did not know of Dunn, but after I explained to them his views on the stone at Abu Rawash and his conclusion that large-scale machinery was responsible for such cutting, several others remarked that Dunn's conclusions were incredulous and that the matter had been settled by the research of University of Manchester professor Denys A. Stocks (2003), as described in his book *Experiments in Egyptian Archaeology: Stoneworking Technology in Ancient Egypt*. Stocks recreated tools meeting the standards of the tools that have been found in ancient Egypt, or are depicted in their art, and used them to cut stone, etch granite, and create small flasks and pottery. "Case closed" was the general consensus from my Egyptologist friends. No one seemed to be interested that Dunn, a master machinist and engineer, determined that the striations in the stone at Abu Rawash could not have been made with the sorts of tools that Stocks had recreated, and neither were they interested in much else that Dunn had investigated. If Stocks's work is conventional Egyptology's answer to these monumental questions that arise regarding the sheer magnitude and precision of the ancient Egyptian temples, statuary, and art, then it seems that the lack of credibility lies with Stock's supporters and not with Dunn.

I use Dunn's research as only one example of a plethora of similar research and conclusions regarding ancient Egyptian technology. Although sloppiness is certainly indicated in the lack of archeological discipline (for instance, there is no way to know if the stone at Abu Rawash was cut during Egypt's Pharaonic times—but how would any other time make it less unique?), it would seem there are enough instances of similar phenomena present in Egypt to titillate the curiosity of mainstream archaeologists, but apparently, this is not the case.

Typically, if Egyptologists are pestered enough to feel a need to respond to such renegade theories, the result is not pretty. Mark Lehner (1997; Lehner & Cayce, 1974; Lehner, Wetterstrom, Giza Plateau Mapping Project, & Ancient Egypt Research Associates, 2007), one of the world's contemporary authorities on the Giza Plateau, argued with John Anthony West's (1993) and Robert M. Schoch's (2012, 1999) theory on the age of the Great Sphinx. Based on evidence of water erosion, West and Schoch posited that the Great Sphinx was constructed many thousands of years before conventional Egyptology postulates, but Lehner et al. (2007) claimed that West and Schoch have no historical context upon which to make such a claim. Although West and Schoch did not declare any sort of advanced technology was utilized in building the Great Sphinx, they contended it was not built in the Old Kingdom by the Pharaoh Khafra (2558–2532 BC), which is the consensus among mainstream archeologists. Lehner et al. obviously had a point. Researchers who ignore the historical context can make nearly any theory look plausible. But that is clearly not the case with Schoch's work. His meticulous scientific research, generated from a highly intelligent and conventionally educated mind, simply followed the data he had acquired. However, Lehner et al. insisted that conventional wisdom states that seldom, if ever, do things occur in the historical record without a reason or just pop up out of the blue. There is typically a thread to follow that connects events and ideas in some logical and rational manner. In this case there appeared to be none, and in the eyes of the mainstream archeological community, the credibility of Schoch's research was threatened.

Since this debate, however, the ancient site at Göbekli Tepe in Turkey has been attributed to a civilization that may have existed more than 10,000 years ago, which gives credence to the possible existence on the Giza plateau of an advanced culture predating the ancient Egyptian culture. Unlike many of the other alternative researchers cited here, Schoch has extensive academic credentials including a doctoral degree in geology and geophysics from Yale University and is currently (2015) a full-time faculty member at the College of General Studies at Boston University. It is certainly reasonable to assume that he conducted his controversial research using sound scientific methods.

As far as the tenacity of other alternative claims, archeologists in general and Egyptologists in particular tend to ignore theories that do not fall within the rigid systems developed for scientific and archeological research. Many elements are taken into consideration before claiming any finding to be truth. Common sense would say, for example, that if an artifact is found that could be constructed using only iron tools, it is not likely to be dated as existing before what is accepted as the dates for the Iron Age. Archeologists simply do not believe that the advancements in technology and culture can move backwards unless the historical context allows them to. This conviction, along with the argument that such construction simply cannot happen according to the laws of physics (such as lifting heavy stones in any manner other than by manpower during an age where only manpower is available), seems to be the primary argument against all of these alternative theories. It is difficult to cite these conclusions, as they do not seem to show up in the record, presumably for much the same reason it would be difficult or impossible to find modern documented record of a serious scientific debate on whether fairies are real or not. However, the analogy of fairies' existence and how 80-ton granite boxes were moved underground 2,500 or so years ago in the Apis bull tombs of Egypt's Saqqara desert without contemporary machinery is not a fair comparison, as the evidence of granite boxes sitting in a real location at which we can see and feel them is quite compelling. Fairies have left no such evidence of their existence.

The political perspective should also be considered in the question of Egypt's national heritage. According to contemporary alternative Egyptologists Robert Bauval and Ahmad Osman (2012), in their book *Breaking the Mirror of Heaven: The Conspiracy to Suppress the Voice of Egypt*, a concerted effort has been made in Egyptian politics, both past and present, to suppress an alternative view of history. Nations are reluctant to alter their national persona, and any new discovery that may diminish their cultural heritage could be disconcerting and is often either ignored or ridiculed and denied further inquiry.

The engineering accomplishments of the ancient Egyptians are nevertheless so noted in modern times that they have almost become caricatures of the Herculean abilities of human beings when they put their minds to accomplishing a challenging task. Adhering to the dictums of the modern scientific method, these works are not looked upon as magical, supernatural, or beyond our current understanding of the universe and the causal powers therein or as requiring any sort of different scientific paradigm to perform. We plainly see the results of these amazing acts—we see the pyramids and the other huge granite structures, temples, and statuary, and although not obvious to our naked eye, we believe the informed reports of Egyptian precision in pyramid block placement, temple stone placement, and other seemingly impossible feats. Modern science, however, does not allow us to go beyond its limitations to explain any of these phenomena, and we fall into *promissory materialism*, which promises us that, one day, materialism will catch up with these anomalies and thus explain them in a way that will not conflict with materialism's established laws.

Still, one thing many of the alternative thinkers have in common with conventional Egyptologists, even those believing in popular extraterrestrial origin theories, is that all that was accomplished in ancient Egypt fits within the materialist Newtonian paradigm of cause-and-effect physics. Much is written today regarding the mystical underpinnings of the ancient Egyptian cosmology, but seldom is it insinuated that the ancient Egyptians moved matter with their minds (sometimes, but seldom!) or that their psyches were somehow capable of manipulating matter in the material world. These ideas seem so extreme, they are not often suggested or brought into serious discussion.

My own personal experiences with the questions presented here regarding the unsolvable mysteries of ancient Egypt include my trip underground to visit the bull sarcophagi of the Serapeum in the Saqqara desert as described in Chapter 1. I also visited Dunn's stone in Abu Rawash. In the first days of my second trip to Egypt in 2005 with my wife, Cindy, we asked our amenable tour guide Amr if we could venture out on a special, possibly forbidden, excursion. Amr, in his typically Egyptian exuberance, said he surely could accommodate our request.

The following day, we arose early and met an employee of Amr's, Mohammad, and our usual driver to set out on our adventure. Sure enough, Abu Rawash was forbidden. Amr gave instructions to Mohammad to at least attempt to procure granted passage to the site. So, on our wobbly trek through the dirt roads of the periphery of Giza, we made our way to some sort of official offices housed in a small clay-brick building on the outskirts of town.

Mohammad went in to negotiate a sanctioned journey while Cindy and I waited under a small tree shading the front entrance to the building—the van was far too warm to occupy when it wasn't moving. As we milled about we attempted to make friends with a feral dog. This turned out to be quite a reckless pursuit, as the small, dirty-white animal almost took a chunk out of my outstretched hand. His aggressive behavior set the tone for this place, and we lingered in the front courtyard while waiting for Mohammad with hands in pockets being eyed by several men with ominous side arms strapped tight about their skinny waists, their dark eyes flashing looks of obvious mistrust. No one seemed to be particularly happy we were there. Most Egyptians, until now, were almost excessively kind, good natured, and eager to engage with tourists. These men seemed to represent a bit of the real Egypt, not the glitzy touristy Egypt in the cities and close to the monuments where being overly courteous could garner a few Egyptian pounds as tips.

After what seemed to be an interminable length of time, Mohammad walked out of the small building toward the van. He said nothing as he walked, with his head slightly bowed. I started to say something to him, and he shook his head with almost imperceptible movement without making eye contact. I took the hint and quietly followed him into the van. We got back onto the road and headed off. Mohammad sat silent for several minutes, then finally turned to us and said, "They did not give us permission, but we go anyway." The driver smiled—even though he wore heavy dark glasses, you could tell his eyes twinkled. "We go anyway," Mohammed repeated.

Cindy and I weren't sure what to think, but we were game for the adventure. My thoughts returned to the men in the courtyard with the dark, suspicious eyes and the guns hanging from their hips. I wondered too if we would run into any more angry desert dogs. Mohammad turned to face the front and said that he had called Amr to get some advice while trying to convince the authorities they should grant us permission to go to the site. Amr had said he would call Zahi Hawass himself if he needed to. Obviously, he decided against that ploy. Zahi Hawass is considered the most "important Egyptologist" of our time—that appellation given to him due more than likely to his celebrity status appearances on countless documentaries on Egypt and his rather outspoken public voice, than on anything to do with Egyptology. Hawass had become the "Lord of the Giza Plateau," allowing nothing to pass by his intense surveillance over the region. He was then Secretary General of the Supreme Council of Antiquities, later Minister of Antiquities, but lost that post during the fall of the Mubarak regime in 2011. He was later invited back by the new government, and then mysteriously quit. Some say he again got the sack.

The site was only about 5 miles from Giza, but the drive seemed endless. Mostly dirt roads, sometimes barely discernable, led us deeper and deeper into the desert. The landscape was not without various outcroppings of civilization, mostly in the form of radio towers or militaristic structures low to the ground with small windows and surrounded by razor-wire fences. At one point, we came upon a sign that said, "Do Not Enter—Military Zone." Our driver glanced at Mohammad as we left the sign in a plume of dust. Mohammad shrugged and tittered nervously.

Finally, we reached our destination, Abu Rawash. It is considered by mainstream Egyptology to be the site of the pyramid of Khufu's son, Djedefre, purported to be a black sheep of the family. Originally, it was thought to be an unfinished pyramid, but recently the consensus has shifted to proclaim that it was in fact finished; however, for some unknown reason, the majority of the structure is mysteriously missing. The jury is still out, however, and many still contend it was never completed. The construction of this pyramid is a bit different than its more popular brethren 5 miles south. A lot of granite was apparently used, and the site is littered with large pieces of the rock in various forms of refinement. Some are carved into compelling shapes for some special use and others are just rough cuts of stone scattered about in various places, now reminiscent of bodies left to decay on a battlefield.

We came to find the inexplicable slab of stone that Chris Dunn had spent so many hours investigating. After about a half hour of periphery exploration, we found the stone, sitting in the same position that Dunn had described, propped up on some smaller stones, looking like a small picnic table ready to be decked out with a desert banquet. I pondered what it would have been like to discover a stone like this in the middle to late part of the 19th century—a seemingly smooth cut of red granite, a slab nearly 4 feet by 3 feet in size, sitting unpretentiously in the desert sun, or wherever it may have been sitting 150 years ago. Upon closer examination, those early explorers would have possibly noticed the faint scratches in the stone, passing in a single line from one side of the slab to the next, stacked one on top of the other like record grooves in vinyl. But who knew what a vinyl record was at the time, which was not in wide use until the 1920s? Why would Petrie, if he had examined this stone in 1883 (he did look over the Abu Rawash pyramid during his stay in Egypt), even notice something unusual about it if no one of his time had yet cut a stone with a large (over 30 feet in diameter) circular saw? Perhaps, and maybe more than likely, no one even noticed.

I set about taking numerous photographs and fell into a deep pondering over the stone. I am not an engineer and knew nothing of what the rows of grooves could mean or imply. However, even with little knowledge of engineering or of ancient stone masonry techniques, I did find the grooves curious and oddly modern in nature. They distinctly appeared as if they were created by one graceful repetitive action, rather than a result of chipping away with diorite stones, small handheld copper saws, or wooden hammers, the alleged tools of the time. What do they say about Occam's Razor?—the solution with the fewer assumptions is usually the correct solution. It seemed a large saw would be the least complicated explanation for what I was observing, without factoring in the historical context. Of course, a large saw in ancient Egypt would be found at the wrong place, in the wrong time—and where was extant evidence of the actual saw?

A howling pack of wild dogs broke my reverie. They were a bit of a distance away, perched on a small hill just downwind from the pyramid complex. Although they were far away, it was clear they were annoyed we had violated their territory. More angry dogs. There were about six of them in the pack, gathering the courage to confront us directly. Mohammad and our driver were tossing stones at them, which never got very close to hitting them. They did stay back, however; at least long enough for us to get ourselves back into the van and rumble down the hill toward the road. As we looked back, we could see the dogs through our wake of dust, running, almost dancing, through the rubble—the jackals of the pyramids protecting the spirits of their ancient overseers.

Most ineffable mysteries of ancient Egypt can be classified in one of two categories—weight or precision. Possibly a third category, but one that is not as popular, would be just plain mystical. The mystical category is difficult to relate to anything concrete, and if it is, regarding pyramid texts, stories, myths, gods, and the like, it is usually not perceived as anything altogether unusual. Any "supernatural" interpretation put on such things would be more than likely considered by mainstream Egyptology to be sensational and incredulous. We can also lump into this category any of the theories that involve pre-Egyptian cultures and civilizations whose peoples may have built the pyramids and Great Sphinx, among other artifacts that have often been suggested not to be of Egyptian origin.

The first two categories of the ineffable mysteries of ancient Egypt, weight and precision, are material and thus have physical evidence to support them. Lots of things we find in the Egyptian desert are very heavy, and much of the controversy that exists today lies in how these heavy things were quarried, shaped, transported, and put into their final positions. The precision category includes anything that required more than primitive reasoning and execution: for example, the mathematics and relationships with the cosmos and other ancient sites throughout the world surrounding the placement and construction of the pyramids, the temples of Luxor, and virtually all of the major monuments. Precision also is found in the microcosm of ancient Egyptian artifacts, the statuary and its near-perfect symmetry, the granite sarcophagi of the Serapeum and its near-perfect right angles and smooth flat surface that rivals today's laser-polished perfection, to name only a few out of the thousands of examples. It would take hundreds of pages to present and attempt to explain these amazing instances of perfect precision. Ancient Egypt's history is filled with these unexplained anomalies, too many to ignore, but many *are* ignored or explained away by conventional Egyptology in highly suspect ways.

Conventional Egyptologists, of course, do have their explanations for many of these phenomena, but not for all of them, and certainly many of these explanations fall short of plausibility or even credibility. The alternative camp's offerings are not much more believable, ranging from extraterrestrial intervention to giant saws powered by some mysterious source. But at times, quite often, it does seem that these more far-fetched explanations are closer to explaining what we see and touch. As mentioned before, one thing all of these clarifications have in common, from the conservative to the radical, is that they are material solutions. They all fall into the realm of Newtonian cause-and-effect physics. What if the explanation for all that is presented here was not materialist? What if the causation for the construction of pyramids, temples, art, statuary, was of the mind and spirit and not of anything mechanical—or at least not wholly mechanical?

This book focuses on the cosmology of ancient Egypt because this ancient yet sophisticated civilization seems to have possessed some unique qualities not as easily observed in other ancient civilizations. It could be argued that many ancient civilizations possess similar attributes, and it has even been suggested that the ancient Egyptian culture may have risen out of the Mayan culture, an entire continent and ocean away (Le Plongeon, 1983), but Egypt is unique in many regards. One particularly important factor in considering ancient Egypt as the culture of focus in this book is the extensive research that has been applied to some of the more esoteric theories behind the creation of the monuments and temples still standing. Although the alternative research on other sites in Bolivia, Peru, and other parts of the world is catching up, concentration is centered here, in Egypt, on these amazing structures, art, statuary and the mysteries surrounding their design and construction primarily to emphasize the effectiveness of the ancient Egyptians' spiritual beliefs in manifesting such physical intricacy and Herculean effort. As far as we can tell, they did not have at their disposal modern tools and machinery and therefore had to accomplish these ineffable feats in some other manner. Even if we adhere to the conventional theories regarding the method in which these structures were designed and built, we still must factor in an amazing dedication to an inner determination and intention the designers and builders more than likely possessed in order to accomplish these feats of construction.

Ancient Egyptian cosmology was expressed not only in their material endeavors but also in their medicine, spiritual life, and even their everyday living. Of these things we know little when compared with all that there is to know about the ancient Egyptian life, and even the existing body of knowledge does not clearly address the psyche-to-matter problem that is at the crux of this book's presentation. In an effort to avoid a certain dualistic perception, it is imperative that not only material considerations be observed with regard to Egyptian sacred science (discussed in detail in the following chapter). The intended application of this book, however, is for a psychotherapy patient to exercise a newfound psychic and spiritual awareness not by building a temple or a pyramid or following some Egyptian spiritual ritual but, instead, by acquiring a deeper understanding of all things real, including, with equal consideration, the inner world of images, story, and symbols in order to assimilate a sacred science into their lives.

References

Bauval, R., & Osman, A. (2012). *Breaking the mirror of heaven: The conspiracy to suppress the voice of ancient Egypt*. Rochester, VT: Bear.

Budge, E. A. W. (1899a). *Egyptian magic*. London, England: Paul.

Budge, E. A. W. (Trans.). (1899b). *The book of the dead: The papyrus of Ani in the British Museum*. London, England: British Museum/Longmans.

Dunn, C. (1998). *The Giza power plant: Technologies of ancient Egypt*. Santa Fe, NM: Bear.

Dunn, C. (2008, July 1). Mega saws of the pyramid builders. *Atlantis Rising*, 32–65.

Judge, W. Q. (1951). *Practical occultism: From the private letters of William Q. Judge*. Pasadena, CA: Theosophical University Press.

Le Plongeon, A. (1983). *The origin of the Egyptians*. Los Angeles, CA: Philosophical Research Society.

Lehner, M. (1997). *The complete pyramids*. New York, NY: Thames.

Lehner, M., & Cayce, E. (1974). *The Egyptian heritage: Based on the Edgar Cayce readings*. Virginia Beach, VA: A.R.E. Press.

Lehner, M., Wetterstrom, W., Giza Plateau Mapping Project, & Ancient Egypt Research Associates. (2007). *Giza reports: The Giza Plateau Mapping Project*. Boston, MA: Ancient Egypt Research Associates.

Maspero, G. (1912). *Art in Egypt* (E. Lee, Trans.). New York, NY: Scribner's.

Napoleon and the Great Pyramid: Myth and reality. (2014). Retrieved from http://www.strangehistory.net/2013/12/02/napoleon-and-the-great-pyramid/

Napoleon I, E. o. t. F., Jomard, M., Lelorgne de Savigny, M. J. C. s., & Fourier, J. B. J. b. (1809–1829). *Description de l'Egypte: Ou recueil des observations et des recherches qui ont été faites en Égypte pendant l'expédition de l'armée française* [Description of Egypt, or the collection of observations and research which were made in Egypt during the expedition of the French Army] (23 vols.). Paris, France: Impériale.

Napoleon's visit to the Great Pyramid. (2014). Retrieved from http://www.gizapyramid.com/history.htm

Ryan, C. J. (1911). The new Egyptology and the theosophical records. *Theosophical Path, 1*(1), 15–19.

Ryan, C. J. (1939). *What is theosophy? A general view for inquirers*. Point Loma, CA: Theosophical University Press.

Schoch, R. M. (with McNally, R. A.). (1999). *Voices of the rocks: A scientist looks at catastrophes and ancient civilizations*. New York, NY: Harmony Books.

Schoch, R. M. (2012). *Forgotten civilization: The role of solar outbursts in our past and future*. Rochester, VT: Inner Traditions.

Stocks, D. A. (2003). *Experiments in Egyptian archaeology: Stoneworking technology in Ancient Egypt*. London, England: Routledge.

Tingley, K. A. W. (1992). *The Gods await*. Pasadena, CA: Theosophical University Press.

West, J. A. (1993). *Serpent in the sky: The high wisdom of ancient Egypt*. Wheaton, IL: Quest Books.

3

WHAT IS SACRED SCIENCE?

The preceding chapter provided a brief overview of the early days of Egyptology and how Napoleon Bonaparte's late-18th-century invasion of Egypt brought European sensibilities to the study of the region. I also briefly investigated a few examples of ancient Egyptian advanced technology from an alternative history perspective. Egyptologists today continue to be confounded by a culture that is largely perceived as primitive yet is one that has obviously created, with astounding precision and efficacy, some of the world's most impressive monuments, statuary, and works of art. I have maintained focus on these tangible artifacts in order to illustrate the connection between a nonmaterialist cosmology, which the ancient Egyptians seemed to possess, and the manifestation of material form. If the mainstream conjectures regarding the method of manufacture of these tangible artifacts does not live up to intense scrutiny (obviously, the mainstream believes they do), it would suggest other sources of energy or, from a more metaphysical perspective, other sources of psychic ability or subjective intention, connectedness, awareness, or consciousness that would allow them to manipulate matter in the obvious way that they did. I believe that Schwaller de Lubicz (1961/1988) and others (Malkowski, 2007; Naydler, 1994, 1996) have described this unique perspective of reality as *sacred science*.

I do not mean to imply that the ancient Egyptians performed these amazing feats of physical manifestation simply by imagining something in their heads (although, theoretically, that is a possibility). I am, however, suggesting that perhaps their unique perspective of reality through sacred science allowed them to do things that have been considered, in our current materialist worldview, as only attainable through mechanized and materialist methods. I again emphasize the material here because it is tangible, and we can examine extant examples of it. The other nonmaterial aspects of their lives were undoubtedly also affected by this perspective. It is, however, very difficult to ascertain these aspects due to the scant records left by the early Egyptians. The central thrust of this book is to examine how an assimilation of this perspective, or cosmology, can help psychotherapy patients achieve the quality of experiences they wish to achieve in their lives. Although the manipulation of the material world is a challenge we all face every day, the point of this proposed assimilation is not to build material monuments, cut stone, or create near symmetrical statuary, but instead to melt down the boundary between the inner world and the material world and to come to an understanding that there is, in fact, no boundary at all. As Carl Jung (1966/1929) said, "presumably the psyche does not trouble itself about our categories of reality; for it, everything that *works* is real" (p. 52). My belief is that, once this false boundary is relinquished, we will live in a world more in harmony with our inner wisdom and thus experience more fulfillment, happiness, purpose, meaning, and peace.

So what is sacred science? Although the modern dictionary definitions of *sacred* and *science* are obviously, by nature, not sufficient to adequately convey the meaning of the term, it is still useful to ponder these textbook definitions for a better understanding of their deeper meanings. The *Oxford Advanced American Dictionary* defines *science* as "knowledge about the structure and behavior of the natural and physical world, based on facts that you can prove, for example by experiments" ("Science," 2011, def. 1). The same resource defines *sacred* as "connected with God or a god; considered to be holy" ("Sacred," 2011, def. 2). *Sacred science* then denotes, according to this narrow dictionary definition, knowledge of the physical and material world as seen through a divine lens—in other words, the holy physical world as it is connected to the divine, to God, or to the gods. To Schwaller de Lubicz, who used the term in the context most relevant to this book, sacred science was not so much a practice but rather a description of the innate intelligence within the human being to know nature wholly from within. This is the consciousness of the heart I have been discussing in previous chapters. The efforts of the individuals who are aware of this innate quality of knowledge then are directed toward creating an outer, material world that is in harmony with this inner wisdom of natural "rightness."

Considering my own broad definition of *soul* presented later in this book, sacred science then could be viewed as a *science with soul*. If all things and nonthings have soul, then the *practice* of sacred science would have to be a practice based in a conscious awareness of the sacredness, or soulfulness, of whatever was being considered. Science is, as defined herein, a knowledge of things, as all things and nonthings possess information that can be known, and sacred science is the inclusion of the holy, or the divine (the innate intelligence of the heart), with that process of knowing. I make an important personal assumption here that the consciousness of the heart that Schwaller was describing considers soul, as I define it, an operator or catalyst that allows the heart a free and unfettered expression of this sacred science.

The interconnectivity displayed by a knowledge of information beyond our own empirical experience suggests that the concept of unity consciousness is important to consider here as well. Although not fundamentally a part of the

Egyptian spiritual paradigm, unity consciousness is implied in later texts attributed to ancient Egypt, most notably the *Corpus Hermeticum* (Lachman, 2011). The ancient Egyptians did, however, see the world, both inner and outer, as part of a divine plan. The outer world was a reflection of that plan, and the efforts made in the outer world were to reflect as accurately as possible the perfect order of the inner world (Naydler, 1996, pp. 96–97). This reflection of the inner, then, was the divine, holy, or sacred nature of the outer world. The material expression in which the Egyptians engaged was infused with what they considered the rightness of their inner world and this inner world's system.

In our modern era, it is not necessary to use the same schema of symbols, myths, and stories the ancient Egyptians used but only to give this inner world the same credence the ancient Egyptians gave theirs, or at least as much as we are capable of giving, considering our current more complete understanding of the information contained within material things. The expression of the inner divine plan, or sacred science, then becomes, in a more contemporary sense, materialism with soul—a paradigm wherein the material world is real and is integrated with an awareness of the mysterious, nonmaterial, rightness of the inner world. Exactly how this integration takes place is not clear, at least not in all situations (for example, currently this integration may be easier to see in the arts than in medical science or engineering). It is necessary only to recognize a possible advantage in attempting to infuse soul into everything we encounter in our current experience—thus making our own relationship with the material world a sacred science. Referring back to the words of Marie-Louise von Franz (1992), "Can matter mirror the psyche?" (p. 18). In the ancient Egyptian world, this mirroring very well may have been an everyday, quite conscious occurrence.

If we were to emulate this ancient Egyptian spiritual cosmology, we would have to make an effort toward making our outer world more harmonious with the rightness of our divine inner world. In our modern times, science is king, but it is not perceived as a sacred science, as the ancient Egyptians perceived their science. As mentioned before, all science (and art), in ancient Egypt was sacred. Medicine, geometry, architecture, astronomy, it was all infused with spirit and spirits—with soul. Sacredness, in this context, is conveyed in the honoring of the unseen, inner, world. Sacredness is found in becoming one with all that is, including the images, ideas, energies, and power that seemingly reside internally in our own psyches and inner world as expressions of the intelligence of the heart. In ancient Egypt, credence was given equally to this inner world and the material world; in fact, the term *equally* implies dualism, and the ancient Egyptian was not aware of any line or separation between this inner world—the world of the gods as innate knowledge—and the outer world of physical manifestation. In a materially oriented culture, a clear distinction exists between what is considered *real*—physical, material, existence—and what is not real—dreams, images, gods, magic, and anything else that occupies the inner world of being.

Gary Lachman (2000), in an article written for the Theosophy Society's journal, *Quest*, commented:

> Schwaller believed ancient Egypt was based on this inner knowing, very unlike our own outer-oriented one. The ancient Egyptians, he argued, were aware of the limitations of purely cerebral consciousness, the Set mind that "granulates" experience into fragments of time and space and is behind our increasing abuse of nature and of each other. Granulated experience produces our familiar world of disconnected things, each a kind of "island reality." ("Functional Consciousness," para. 3)

The "limitations" that Lachman says the Egyptians acknowledged have compounded in our modern culture to a point where they not only threaten our own personal fulfillment of life but also threaten our very existence. How do we begin to free ourselves from these limitations?

Jeremy Naydler (1996), in *Temple of the Cosmos: The Ancient Egyptian Experience of the Sacred*, suggested that we, as a modern culture, cannot and should not embrace Egyptian sacred science and spirituality in a literal way. He explained:

> Our modern consciousness is not the same as the ancient consciousness. It has been through a long developmental process that we should honor. Simply to embrace ancient Egyptian spirituality today would be to deny the very meaning implicit in the extraordinary historical process that is the cultural biography of the West. The importance of ancient Egypt today lies in its being a reminder that our modern culture has deeper roots than we may have suspected, deeper not only historically but also spiritually. In tapping these roots we go to a profound source of inspiration and guidance. (p. xi)

It does seem to be possible, however, at least to begin the work toward a serious integration of this unique paradigm within our current materialist perspective. Dissolving the line of dualism between the inner world and the outer reality would be difficult; in fact, it would more than likely take many generations of psychic evolution even to begin to come close to such a way of being. Nevertheless, in certain areas of our culture, it may be less problematic to begin this process in a meaningful way. Art and the role of the artist come to mind immediately. Artists in our culture are probably the closest to embracing this way of being; however, our culture's view of art is clearly dualist, as it does not afford art the same place of importance as useful and productive expressions of materialism. Although artists may be ensconced in a way of life with a more integrated worldview, the difficulty of functioning and creating within a culture that does not share this view has great impact on the quality, intention, and meaning of their art. Another area that seems obvious as a place to venture into this integration of the inner and outer world is psychotherapy.

According to Robert Bauval's (1999) research, all activities of the ancient Egyptians were forms of sacred science. Although the majority of Bauval's continuing investigation involves a search for hidden chambers and passageways in the Giza Plateau complex, he presented many ideas, theories, and interpretations of

Egyptology in his report on the Great Pyramid, *Secret Chamber: The Quest for the Hall of Records*. Most notably, Bauval pulls his readers away from a purely scientific and objective analysis of Egyptian facts and figures and lures them toward a more mystical and spiritual perspective.

In one profound example, Bauval cited German engineer Rudolf Gantenbrink's pioneering work on the so-called airshafts of the King's Chamber of the Great Pyramid. Gantenbrink had designed and constructed a small robotic device whose specific purpose was to crawl up the small openings in the chamber with a light and camera to explore what was to be seen. Partially up one of the shafts, a mysterious obstruction was found, which came to be called *Gantenbrink's Door*. Bauval quoted a report from Gantenbrink describing his work in purely scientific terms of measurement, objective analysis, and the like. Bauval commented on Gantenbrink's effort:

> This is like trying to find the soul of a person by dissecting his body. Sadly, this is the very thing that has been happening to the scholarship of ancient Egypt—and indeed to other ancient cultures—when left in the hands of "scientists" alone. Egyptology is not a "science," it is a *sacred science*. (1999, p. 53)

Bauval expressed his hope for a study of Egyptology that includes a more inner-world and soul-felt perspective, which requires ranking the unseen in importance equal to the seen and observable.

The Orion Mystery, by Bauval and historian Adrian Gilbert (1994), tells a similar story but focuses specifically on some of the alternative history theories and discoveries made regarding the Giza pyramid complex. The authors discussed the conventional history of the pyramids as described by modern Egyptologists and then offered alternative ideas about their history and function, including insights regarding the purpose of the shafts found in the King's and Queen's chambers as well as thoughts regarding the alignment of the three pyramids with the stars of Orion's belt. Although most of Bauval's work does not focus on religious and spiritual aspects of ancient Egyptian cosmology, he does present alternative ideas that support a less materialist foundation of Egyptian cosmology. As previously noted, Bauval's understanding of the unique Egyptian spiritual perspective is thorough, and his work clearly reflects this awareness.

Bauval teamed up with another prominent alternative Egyptian history scholar, Graham Hancock, in writing *The Message of the Sphinx* (Hancock & Bauval, 1996). Much emphasis in this work is placed on the ancient Egyptians' acumen with regard to the study of the heavens and how the star field they observed relates to the land and the buildings placed on it. Again, the pyramid complex and its correlation with the stars are presented as evidence of the ancient Egyptians' uncanny knowledge of astronomy and their effort to integrate the heavens with their earthly, material existence. Bauval and Hancock indicated that the Egyptians' ground plans for the Giza Plateau—with the placement of the pyramids, the Great Sphinx, and the so-called airshafts in the great pyramid, among many other considerations—all suggest profound religious and cosmological foundations. They professed that these ideas "express the philosophy 'as above, so below' and advocated the drawing down to earth of cosmic powers as an essential step in Mankind's quest for knowledge of the divine and immortality of the soul" (p. 132). They correlated this intention with the wishes of Hermes as indicated in the *Corpus Hermeticum*.

John Anthony West's (1993) seminal work, *Serpent in the Sky*, presents similar alternative Egyptology concepts. Early in his illustrious career, West was an associate professor of natural science. He is probably best known for his research on the Giza Plateau and his conclusion that the Great Sphinx as well as possibly the pyramids themselves predate conventional Egyptology's supposed dates of the creation of the Egyptian culture (the dynastic period being estimated as beginning between 3300 BCE and 3200 BCE, according to White, 1970, p. 138). West asserted as well that no distinction could be made between the ancient Egyptians' conception of *science* and what they called *religion*:

> In Egypt, art, science, philosophy and religion were aspects or facets of a complete understanding, and were employed simultaneously: there was no Egyptian art without science, no philosophy that was not religious. Central to this complete understanding was the knowledge that man, through his faculties and physique, represented the created image of all creation. And Egyptian symbolism and all measures were therefore simultaneously scaled to man, to the earth, and ultimately to the solar system. (p. 69)

It is clear from this statement that West was heavily influenced by the work of R. A. Schwaller de Lubicz, as he cited Schwaller's comments about symbolism ultimately being scaled to man, the earth, and the cosmos. Also notable is West's distinction that not only was spirituality present in science but science was also present in spirituality.

We have already become well acquainted with R. A. Schwaller de Lubicz's work and influence. As mentioned earlier, he is considered by many in the field of Egyptian esoterica to be the father of this concept of ancient Egyptian sacred science. His primary fieldwork took place at the Luxor Temple complex in Upper Egypt. The resulting study was a gargantuan consolidation of those 15 years that Schwaller and his wife, Isha, performed in the desert sands of Egypt. *The Temple of Man: Apet of the South at Luxor* (1957/1998) comprises two volumes containing more than 1,000 oversized pages of narrative, mathematical figures, and drawings of detailed images of Egyptian art, maps, temple layouts, and other architectural renderings. The mass of information and attention to detail that this work encompasses is difficult even to begin to assimilate. Although considered today by most mainstream Egyptologists to be esoteric and contrary to the more conventional results of modern archeological study, Schwaller's work is of utmost importance to the alternative and esoteric ancient Egyptian researcher.

R. A. Schwaller de Lubicz was born René Adolphe Schwaller in 1887 in Alsace-Lorraine, at the time a part of Germany. His father was a well-to-do pharmacist, and

Schwaller did develop a keen interest in chemistry after completing an apprenticeship with his father and moving on to Paris to study chemistry and physics some time in his late teens. There he acquired a love for alchemy, which stayed with him and informed his life's work. The young Schwaller apparently was quite an exceptional scholar and dedicated seeker of knowledge and enlightenment. He fervently studied ancient texts of alchemy from the 13th and 14th centuries. He even became interested in art and studied painting with the famed impressionist Henri Matisse for a time in the early 20th century. Here, Schwaller began to formulate the most important perceptions of his life. Matisse was working acutely with color in an effort not only to recreate the material representation of the subjects of his paintings but to capture their spiritual essence as well—with a material conveyance in the colors of paint on a canvas. Schwaller saw in Matisse, and in his work with him, that metaphysical awareness was impossible to achieve without some suggestion of the physical and that the physical cannot exist without a metaphysical base. This is the foundation of sacred science—psyche to matter and, simultaneously, matter to psyche; a reality cannot be whole without both perceptions fully integrated.

Through his work with the famous impressionist at L'Académie Matisse, Schwaller became thoroughly familiar with the ideas of Henri Bergson by attending his lectures at the Sorbonne. Bergson was a passionate philosopher popular for a time, writing and lecturing on his beliefs that direct experience, intuition, and the manner in which a person processes these phenomena has a more imperative connection to reality than science and rationalism alone. Bergson, without being aware of Schwaller's later invention of the terms, was speaking of the consciousness of the heart in concurrence with the consciousness of the intellect. Combining his experiences with Matisse, his own personal studies in alchemy and the origin of matter, and his absorption of Bergson's philosophy, Schwaller was building a powerful cosmology of his own. Through these deep passions in philosophy and alchemy, Schwaller aspired to learn the true nature of matter and how consciousness relates to it.

After a brief stint in the military as a chemist during World War I, Schwaller adopted the nom de plume *Aor*, which means *Light of the Higher Mind*, and wrote articles and journals on social reform, the implementation of peace, and the universal laws of harmony. It was during this time that he met Oscar Vladislas de Lubicz Milosz, a Lithuanian mystic and poet with whom Schwaller felt close enough to share his Hermetic philosophy. Schwaller was instrumental in helping Milosz to secure Lithuanian independence, and in 1919, as a gesture of gratitude and appreciation, Milosz bestowed upon him his family name of de Lubicz.

In 1922, Schwaller and his closest group of friends left France for Switzerland. They settled in the small town of St. Moritz in the Swiss Alps. Here they created the Station Scientifique Suhalia, an institution complete with laboratory equipment, forges, an observatory, a printing press, and even looms. Schwaller immersed himself in a community of like-minded individuals—artists, artisans, scholars, philosophers, and craftsmen—all dedicated to a contemplative way of life through creation, discussion, and writing. Schwaller even practiced the art and science of applied alchemy and created uniquely colored glass artifacts based on ancient formulae that had not been successfully replicated since their original creation 600 years before. Through these associations and activities he continued to develop the worldview and philosophy that prepared him for the pinnacle of his life's work in Egypt.

Schwaller also came under the influence of several of the pioneers of quantum physics—Max Planck, Niels Bohr, Werner Heisenberg, and Albert Einstein. No doubt the work of these men informed Schwaller's theosophical foundation and allowed him to make connections with science, physical realities, and the teachings of ancient cultures. One of Schwaller's most important principles in his cosmology is the tense yet illuminating effect of intelligent comprehension united with heartfelt awareness. Quantum physics' uncertainty principle, as developed by Werner Heisenberg in 1927, posits that one cannot know simultaneously the position and the speed of a subatomic particle. This notion suggests an illogical concept of holding mutually exclusive ideas together at the same time. Carl Jung had discussed a similar concept he called *tension of the opposites*, based on the conflict between opposites creating pressure in the alchemical vessel (Jung, 1953–1979). It is in this tension, this state of holding two opposing concepts together in simultaneous awareness, that the divine is found.

Gary Lachman (2000) observed:

> This "simultaneity of opposite states" plays a great part in Schwaller's understanding of Egyptian hieroglyphics. It characterizes what he calls *symbolique*, a way of holding together the object of sense perception and the content of inner knowing, in a kind of creative polarity. When the Egyptians saw the hieroglyph of a bird, he argued, they knew it was a sign for the actual, individual creature, but they also knew it was a symbol of the "cosmic function" that the creature exemplified—flight—as well as all the myriad characteristics associated with it. Hieroglyphics did not merely designate; they evoked. ("Science and Theosophy," para. 4)

Probably the most powerful influence in Schwaller's life and work was his interest in and study of alchemy. Due to his early training as a scientist and chemist, Schwaller was able to integrate hard material science with the lofty world of spirit and transcendent thought. For example, he rejected Carl Jung's ideas that alchemy was a purely psychic device that had little to do with the material world. Schwaller believed alchemy to be a practice that not only transformed the consciousness of the alchemist but also manipulated physical matter.

In 1936, on the prompting of his wife Isha, Schwaller headed for Egypt, and there he had a revelation that, in the desert sands of this ancient country, he would find the answers to the questions that perplexed him regarding the evolution of consciousness. He remained there until 1951, researching primarily the Luxor Temple complex. The essence of his conclusions at Luxor play a crucial role in understanding the importance of the inner imaginal world as an integral part of the ancient Egyptians' reality and architectural science. According to Schwaller's findings, the ancient Egyptians were capable of creating precision beyond what is considered possible for an ancient civilization of this time—and only possible with what Schwaller called a clear and functioning "intelligence of the heart." In other words, the work that researchers such as Christopher Dunn have shown us, the manipulation of gargantuan, hard stone coerced into the symmetry and precision accomplished by the ancient Egyptians, could not have been executed without what Schwaller has described as intelligence of the heart.

As Schwaller related his move from the material perspective of nature to a more nonmaterial paradigm, he described what he found to be this intelligence of the heart, or consciousness of the heart. He outlined a form of conscious evolution that could be the foundation, as this book suggests, for an informed methodology in psychotherapy that not only honors the material world but also views the inner innate knowledge all mankind possesses as an active and vital participant in an individual's navigation through life. Consciousness of the heart is independent of the information received by the material senses and forms the vastness of the entirety of life. Schwaller posited two types of intelligence: cerebral intelligence, which is represented by the symbol; and the intelligence of the heart, represented, for example, by the ancient Egyptian hieroglyph, which goes beyond a symbolic[1] representation of information to convey the innate quality of the intelligence of the heart.

This concept of hieroglyphs having meaning that goes beyond mere symbolism is illustrated elegantly by Robert Bauval's description of the meaning behind the hieroglyph for the wagtail bird, found in his book *Secret Chamber: The Quest for the Hall of Records*. Here, Bauval described the innate qualities that lie within the hieroglyph. The little Egyptian sign, he said, represents not only the wagtail bird but also the entirety of the experience of the wagtail, and in so doing, represents not just the human experience of the wagtail but also the wagtail's experience and everything within the field of the wagtail, including the seasonal metamorphosis of the creature itself, the experience of the sun whose rays warm the wagtail's eggs and chicks, the entire history of the species, and even aspects of the being of the wagtail that are beyond sensory perception (pp. 50–51).

In an attempt to simplify the difficult concepts found in *The Temple of Man*, in his later book, *The Egyptian Miracle*, Schwaller de Lubicz (1963/1985) reported that one foundation of the Pharaonic mind is "faith in an origin that cannot be situated in time and space" (p. 11). He declared, "This is reality absolute, not to be grasped by our intelligence. This cannot be regarded as a mystery: it is the eternal Present Moment, indivisible Unity" (p. 11). In other words, comprehending a complete and whole reality requires that it be neither split into a duality of mind and matter nor quantified through time and space. The deep connection of numeric meaning and mathematical sacredness and the connection between the Temple of Man and the temple built of stone resting near the Nile in Luxor comprised an essential tenet of Schwaller de Lubicz's assessment of ancient Egyptian cosmology.

In another of his significant works, *Sacred Science*, Schwaller de Lubicz (1961/1988) concluded, "According to the evidence inscribed during a period of over four thousand years, ancient Egypt did not have a 'religion' as such; *it was religion in its entirety*, in the broadest and purest acceptation of the term" (p. 6). This observation is also an example of a primary thrust of this book's inquiry regarding how a civilization that had such spectacular physical triumphs demonstrated in architecture, engineering, medicine, and art could be founded entirely—per modern scholars' assessment—on spirituality, a substance without form.

In a more contemporary setting, Rosemary Clark (2003), a modern Egyptian priestess practicing the ancient arts of Egyptian religious ritual, commented on a modern perspective of sacred science in her set of books, *The Sacred Magic of Ancient Egypt* (2003) and *The Sacred Tradition in Ancient Egypt* (2000). These volumes comprise a practitioner's guide to rituals and the practice of the ancient Egyptian arts. She stated:

> Evidence of Egypt's Sacred Science is abundant—in the design and construction of monuments that cannot be duplicated today, in an elaborate practice of mummification that eludes our understanding, in the record of a superior skill in medicine mingled with magic—to name a few. But even though we can, for instance, intellectually discern examples of advanced geometry in the construction of Egyptian pyramids, or account for the success of their healing art by virtue of the placebo effect, the meaning and objective of these endeavors is quite often eluded. (2003, p. 21)

Clark made an astute point regarding the elusive nature of these feats defying intellectual understanding of their meaning and purpose. Possibly, this missing element, from the ancient Egyptian point of view, would be the unseen force or field that brings objective material reality in direct union with the imaginal, inner, intentional world. As presented throughout this book, the ancient Egyptians understood the harmony between the materially lived world and the world beyond time as an expression of *ma'at*.

The primary objective of Clark's two tomes was to bring back to life the ancient Egyptian ritual and magic in a close-to-literal fashion. She documented rituals, texts, and suggestions for temple construction as well as a myriad of other tools to bring forth the ritualistic procedures as closely as possible to what she perceived were the actual events practiced in ancient times. About her research team's process, Clark stated, "Over a number of years, we reconstructed a protocol of philosophical instruction, art, music, science, design, liturgy, and religious practice that was as close to that of the ancient priesthood as could be realized" (p. xx). She further clarified her approach to the research:

> The worship of the Egyptian deities played no part in this discipline; rather, it defined itself as a repertoire of exploring archetypal images using astrological keys in concert with pharaonic symbolism. The unexpected result of this work was the discovery of an inner temple that could be accessed through this religious practice, a psychic reservoir of information that transmitted itself into our everyday lives. Proof of its nature came in a

> range of phenomena from the emergence of creative skills to spontaneous healings, all confirming that another dimension of experience had been initiated. (p. xx)

Clark demonstrated, through actual practice, the effects of incorporating this Egyptian cosmological paradigm into an individual's daily life.

Clark went on to comment about the possibility of bringing into current culture the enormous success in material expression the ancient Egyptians experienced through "the wisdom to build monuments that will endure for millennia and the insight to coexist harmoniously with the natural environment" (p. 12) and how this could "revolutionize the education, science, religion, and philosophy of our time" (p. 12). She proposed:

> The key to making this prospect a reality is in the rediscovery of what the symbolists call the Sacred Science, a body of knowledge from which all of Egypt's endeavors arose. Through the prodigious studies that [Schwaller] de Lubicz completed—of temples, literature, and art—he revealed that the use of this science was a conscious, deliberate effort to apply the deepest spiritual wisdom to human life. This was effected through the use of what we would today call magic, but which to the Egyptians was a natural technology of transformation. (p. 12)

The key phrase here is "conscious, deliberate effort." The ancient Egyptians evidently practiced their spirituality as they practiced their science, in a deliberate manner rather than as a private sidebar to their daily lives or proselytizing a dogma or belief as being the one and only. Ancient Egyptians simply treated their spiritual world as reality and consulted the laws of that world with the same intention and attention as they consulted the laws of the material world in which they expressed this reality.

Speculative theorist Michael Baigent (2006), in his book *The Jesus Papers*, presented another concept fundamental to the thesis presented in this book. The relationship the ancient Egyptians had with the outer world is mentioned several times throughout these pages, but Baigent contextualized it clearly and succinctly in this passage:

> Coexisting within this universal perfection were two worlds: the physical world, which we are born into and within which we live, and the other world to which we travel when we die, the Duat, or the Far-World. The Far-World was not seen as separate, as some heaven or hell far away from or unconnected with mundane existence. Rather, the Far-Word was ever-present. It was believed to exist simultaneously with the physical world, intertwining with it like the two snakes around the caduceus of Hermes. It was with us all the time even though we could not normally see it or travel to it until we died. (p. 160)

Another important point Baigent made is that the movement in and out of this "Far-World" was literal and not purely psychological. As discussed in further detail in chapters 4 and 7, Carl Jung (1955–1956/1970) publically perceived this alchemical transformation to be primarily psychological and saw only the *consequences* and *results* of this transformation as physical. Marie-Louise von Franz and others have suggested a psyche-to-matter connection but specified it as an acausal connection that is not dependent on linear time, meaning that an inner thought would not be the cause of an outer physical manifestation. The inner and outer worlds are instead seen as linked through meaning and not causality, and if there is a mirroring of sorts between an inner creation and an outer manifestation, it is considered a synchronicity (von Franz, 1980, pp. 78–79). There is much debate surrounding synchronicity and its acausal nature. Cause and effect require a linear time construct, and Einstein (1961), for one, was clear in suggesting that linear time may be an illusion (Bernstein, 1989). As reflected in Jung's *Collected Works* (1953–1979), as his research and writing progressed, he himself changed his mind regarding many earlier postulations. According to various authors and scholars cited in this book as well as the general thesis of this work, the ancient Egyptian paradigm of the transformation or transitioning process is speculated to be both internal and external as well as imaginal and physical.

I cannot complete this chapter on ancient Egyptian sacred science without commenting further on the work of the contemporary philosopher Jeremy Naydler. Naydler's scholarship has contributed enormously to our current understanding of the Egyptian cosmology. A more thorough understanding of Egyptian consciousness of the heart and sacred science and its practical, modern, implications cannot be found in any contemporary literature. He wrote:

> Today we fall short of the kind of awareness of the spirit world that pervaded ancient Egyptian culture. If there was then a recognition of the peculiar capacity of the image or object created by the human hand to provide a physical home for spirit, we, by contrast, have constructed for ourselves a world that rests upon the presupposition that what is material excludes spirit. We fail to see that the objects that we surround ourselves with, and which in some cases accompany us through the day, can mediate spiritual presences. We delude ourselves into thinking that they are simply inanimate. But in the world of the ancient Egyptians there were no "objects" as such: every object was at the same time potentially a subject. Thus paintings and sculptures could become alive, because they formed a living point of contact, a kind of magical juncture, between exterior and interior realities. (2009, p. 130)

To the ancient Egyptian, everything was vibrant with life. Everything that came into awareness, whether it be an internal thought or vision or an external physical manifestation that stimulated the senses, had meaning behind it, and through that meaning, a movement toward a greater harmony was achieved. As Naydler said, in our current materialist culture we do not give the material world spirit and thus see it as essentially dead and inanimate—soulless. It is no wonder that such a large number of us have lost a sense of meaning and purpose.

The focus thus far in this book has been on the physical results (such as the material temple constructions and pyramids of ancient Egypt) of this sacred orientation. Those of us today who find comfort in engaging with the spiritual world very often reject a spirituality presented within a materialist paradigm, thus we are also guilty of a similar prejudice. Our problem lies in a duality perceived between spirit and the material. It would therefore seem that the task at hand would be to find a method to cultivate an awareness of spirit in the material that would bring life and meaning to a world of seemingly dead objects. I have postulated that the ancient Egyptians could and did do this and that it could be reasonably assumed that this sacred orientation was present in all other aspects of ancient Egyptian life. The physical objects such as their monuments, temples, and art are easy to observe and contemplate as they stand in utter magnificence in the vast desert of modern-day Egypt. What is not readily apparent is the precision with which they were built; the deep and exacting intention behind the manner of construction and execution, placement, and precise symmetry; and their evident, almost unerring success in terms of their deeper, and spiritual, meaning and purpose.

What is then described here is a civilization that seemed to understand the relationship between mind and matter, intention and execution. Regarding this acumen, a question is often repeated among alternative and mainstream researchers alike: what was the purpose behind such precision and such exacting nature of their material executions? The ancient Egyptians were aware of the symmetry and harmony of the universe, of all living and nonliving things, and of matter, mind, and imagination. For them, it all worked together as a unity of enactment. Precision was simply the result of this unity and this intention to create harmony with all that is—to see the outer physical work reflect the inner imaginal world in all its perfection.

Let us ponder our current state of affairs: a world that is dying from consumerism and wanton destruction and disregard, its natural processes of ecological stability grossly out of harmony with the intentions and acts of the humans that drain it of life and vibrancy. This is a world where the individual person is lost in mundane confusions and material challenges of ill health, failed relationships, desire for material acquisition, and disconnection from purpose and meaning. What has contemporary humanity lost in the modern materialist paradigm that causes rejection of the unseen, inner world, thus perceiving it as not having any sort of essential meaning? Is it possible that modern materialist cosmology has lost a connection with soul or is absent a consciousness of the heart, as Schwaller de Lubicz described it? We have seen thus far in this book how those in the ancient Egyptian culture kept this consciousness of heart foremost in their thinking and in the execution of their inner thoughts and ideas in the physical realm. In our present time, have we lost all significant connection with what the ancient Egyptians possessed and carried with them first and foremost? How has the abandonment of a consciousness of heart in modern times affected humans' present psychological as well as physical state, considering the present health of this planet, culture, and individual psyches?

These are all difficult questions to contemplate, let alone answer, but an attempt to do so is essential. We may be approaching the end of times as our planet coughs and sputters out its last breaths. If there is a solution to our psychic and physical predicament, it may lie in newly embracing the ancient ways of the Egyptians. Our perception of our own individual experience is a reflection of what we hold within us as beliefs, limitations, and imaginings. If we limit our experiences to only those which a material mechanism can create for us, then we have lost our connection with the soul of the universe. Modern, conventional psychotherapy is concerned primarily with behavior as a result of internal thinking. Depth psychotherapy is concerned primarily with bringing the unconscious into the conscious light in a way that affects our thinking and thus our behavior. Is there a psychotherapy that is concerned primarily with integrating the inner world with the outer world and that strives for harmony with both worlds, as one world? If not, now may be the time to consider it.

Note

1 Schwaller de Lubicz (1951/1978) defined *symbolic* and *symbol* in a unique manner. He believed that symbols represented a process of conveying a very specific, suprarational meaning (past the limitations of a rational system), not merely as representations of conventional description.

References

Baigent, M. (2006). *The Jesus papers: Exposing the greatest cover-up in history*. San Francisco, CA: HarperSanFrancisco.

Bauval, R. (1999). *Secret chamber: The quest for the hall of records*. London, England: Century.

Bernstein, J. (1989, February 27). A critic at large: Besso. *The New Yorker*, pp. 86–94.

Clark, R. (2000). *The sacred tradition in ancient Egypt: The esoteric wisdom revealed*. St. Paul, MN: Llewellyn.

Clark, R. (2003). *The sacred magic of ancient Egypt: The spiritual practice restored*. St. Paul, MN: Llewellyn.

Einstein, A. (1961). *Relativity: The special and the general theory; a popular exposition*. New York, NY: Crown.

Hancock, G., & Bauval, R. (1996). *The message of the Sphinx: A quest for the hidden legacy of mankind*. New York, NY: Crown.

Jung, C. G. (1953–1979). *The collected works of C. G. Jung* (H. Read, M. Fordham, G. Adler, & W. McGuire, Eds.) (R. F. C. Hull, Trans.) (20 vols.). Princeton, NJ: Princeton University Press.

Jung, C. G. (1966). The aims of psychotherapy. In H. Read, M. Fordham, G. Adler, & W. McGuire (Eds.), *The collected works of C. G. Jung* (R. F. C. Hull, Trans.) (Vol. 16, pp. 35–52). Princeton, NJ: Princeton University Press. (Original work published 1929)

Jung, C. G. (1970). Mysterium coniunctionis. In H. Read, M. Fordham, G. Adler, & W. McGuire (Eds.), *The collected works of C. G. Jung* (R. F. C. Hull, Trans.) (Vol. 14). Princeton, NJ: Princeton University Press. (Original work published 1955–1956)

Lachman, Gary (2000, January–February). Rene Schwaller de Lubicz and the intelligence of the heart. *Quest, 89*(1), 4–11. Retrieved from https://www.theosophical.org/publications/quest-magazine/42-publications/quest-magazine/1281-rene-schwaller-de-lubicz-and-the-intelligence-of-the-heart

Lachman, G. (2011). *The quest for Hermes Trismegistus: From ancient Egypt to the modern world.* Edinburgh, Scotland: Floris Books.
Malkowski, E. F. (2007). *The spiritual technology of ancient Egypt: Sacred science and the mystery of consciousness.* Rochester, VT: Inner Traditions.
Naydler, J. (1994). *On the divinity of the Gods.* Oxford, United Kingdom: Abzu.
Naydler, J. (1996). *Temple of the cosmos: The ancient Egyptian experience of the sacred.* Rochester, VT: Inner Traditions.
Naydler, J. (2009). *The future of the ancient world: Essays on the history of consciousness.* Rochester, VT: Inner Traditions.
Sacred. (2011). In *Oxford advanced American dictionary.* Retrieved from http://oaadonline.oxfordlearnersdictionaries.com/dictionary/sacred
Schwaller de Lubicz, R. A. (1978). *Symbol and symbolism* (D. Lawlor & R. Lawlor, Trans.). New York, NY: Autumn Press. (Original work published 1951)
Schwaller de Lubicz, R. A. (1985). *The Egyptian miracle: An introduction to the wisdom of the temple* (A. VandenBroeck & G. VandenBroeck, Trans.). New York, NY: Inner Traditions International. (Original work published 1963)
Schwaller de Lubicz, R. A. (1988). *Sacred science: The king of pharaonic theocracy* (A. VandenBroeck & G. VandenBroeck, Trans.). Rochester, VT: Inner Traditions International. (Original work published 1961)
Schwaller de Lubicz, R. A. (1998). *The temple of man: Apet of the South at Luxor* (2 vols.) (R. Lawlor & D. Lawlor, Trans.). Rochester, VT: Inner Traditions. (Original work published 1957)
Science. (2011). In *Oxford advanced American dictionary.* Retrieved from http://oaadonline.oxfordlearnersdictionaries.com/dictionary/science
von Franz, M.-L. (1980). *Alchemy: An introduction to the symbolism and the psychology.* Toronto, Canada: Inner City Books.
von Franz, M.-L. (1992). *Psyche and matter.* Boston, MA: Shambhala.
West, J. A. (1993). *Serpent in the sky: The high wisdom of ancient Egypt.* Wheaton, IL: Quest Books.
White, J. E. M. (1970). *Ancient Egypt: Its culture and history.* Mineola, NY: Dover.

4

THE PSYCHE-TO-MATTER PROBLEM

What is the psyche-to-matter problem? To start, the problem is a dualist's problem. The notion of dualism is that mind and body exist in two separate realms—the mind being nonphysical and the body, physical. Seventeenth-century philosopher René Descartes is most famous for his assertion that the mind cannot exist outside of the body, and the body cannot think. The "problem" occurs when trying to understand or demonstrate how one realm communicates with the other. How does a nonphysical component affect a physical one? If the nonphysical is purely nonmechanical, how does it manipulate a material object? It is beyond the scope of this book to even briefly investigate the myriad theories and philosophies regarding duality and nonduality in an attempt to solve or even fully understand this problem. However, I will endeavor to illuminate a sampling of ideas that may shed light on the problem as it pertains to ancient Egyptian sacred science and the practice of modern psychotherapy.

The ancient Egyptians most probably did not perceive their universe in a dualistic fashion. To them the reality of form and the reality of nonform functioned together as one, and both had equal credence. Although it is impossible to know for certain, it seems they did not entertain a Cartesian-esque philosophy. If this is true, they did not contemplate the psyche-to-matter problem because, to them, it was not a problem. They would have simply seen their world as one reality, inner and outer, and did not concern themselves with *how* the inner world manipulated the outer, physical world—it just did. Or so it seems, considering the amazing feats that they accomplished beyond what is ostensibly possible for a civilization of their epoch. It may be a stretch for some to assume that the ancient Egyptians may have mastered some form of mind over matter, but considering what we have learned about Schwaller de Lubicz's sacred science and consciousness of the heart, this may be a plausible consideration.

Given our modern dualistic cosmology, if we were to suggest that an image in the mind could somehow produce a material manifestation in the outer world, we would be faced with the psyche-to-matter problem. However, we also would be describing how most human-made creation comes to be. But there are steps in between an idea in the mind and its presentation in material form. Tools are created (which are themselves also ideas first) using the laws of cause-and-effect physics; a mechanism is put into place that then turns the idea into form. We are only limited by the mechanism we have available to us. This is a formidable limitation, as our imagination has always outpaced the supposed mechanism required in order to put an imagined thought into material existence. Take time travel, for example. This idea has been present in the creative mind for quite some time, but the laws of the material universe have limited us when it comes to implementing the tool or mechanism to make it a physical reality. Even the ability of the mind that formulates a thought to move the physical body's musculature in order to make the tool is not fully understood by modern science. You can see how this psyche-to-matter issue can indeed be a problem.

So why not skip the mechanism as well as the limitations of Newtonian physics and just go straight from mind to form? Many say we can (see my discussion of the New Thought movement later in this chapter and in Chapter 6), but this then falls into the realm of parapsychology, metaphysics, spirituality, and magic—or possibly quantum mechanics. The psyche-to-matter problem, according to some, could conceivably be solved by quantum theory. The observer effect may be enough to prove that consciousness alone creates the physical world by collapsing the quantum wave of potential and possibility into the objective and defined material particles that make up a manifest physical reality. Others, possibly including the majority of conventional theoretical physicists, believe the effects of the strange and weird world of quantum particles and wave potentials are confined to the world of atoms and phenomena smaller than atoms. They assume that the big world of big things works just fine without this weirdness, and action within this macrocosm can be predicted with near-perfect accuracy.

The pioneers of quantum physics, including Niels Bohr, Max Planck, Louis de Broglie, Werner Heisenberg, and Albert Einstein, among others, were all rather perplexed by the strange phenomena they were experiencing in their work in the early part of the 20th century. Einstein had a difficult time accepting the theories of quantum physics. He did believe these novel theories were correct, but as they stood at the time they did not make sense to him; the theories did not explain things in their entirety.

Quantum mechanics researchers Bruce Rosenblum and Fred Kuttner (2011), in their book *Quantum Enigma*, sum up both Einstein's concern about quantum theory and the extent of seriousness quantum theory should elicit:

> Einstein was also bothered by the theory's claim that if you observed a small object, an atom, say, to be someplace, it was your *looking* that caused it to be there. Does that apply to big things? In principle, yes. Ridiculing quantum theory, Einstein once asked a fellow physicist, only *half*-jokingly, if he believed the moon was there only when he looked at it. According to

> Einstein, if you took quantum theory seriously, you denied the existence of a physically real world independent of its observation. This is a serious charge. (p. 4)

Rosenblum and Kuttner also delve into some of the more esoteric theories about quantum mechanics and how they may be related to spirituality, metaphysics, and consciousness. This book does not provide a theory about the workings behind spiritual concepts, but what is relevant here is the presentation of modern scientific ideas speculating on the existence of a reality that is not dependent on physical attributes in order to be considered authentic and vital. At the very least, simply being aware of the question can open doors to understanding the importance of these ideas.

Astrobiologist Paul Davies and astrophysicist John Gribbin (2007) offer a clear and easily understood presentation of the matter/nonmatter issue in their book, *The Matter Myth.* These authors submit their ideas on the exact nature of matter and physical reality and expound on current ideas and discoveries relating to quantum physics and the underlying reality of a material world. It is essential to understand what is known about the scientific observation of physical reality before any careful consideration can be made of alternative ideas of reality and whether these alternative ideas have any real meaning in the understanding of the cosmos. Davies and Gribbin posit:

> The matter myth is built on the fiction that the physical Universe consists of nothing but a collection of inert particles pulling and pushing each other like cogs in a deterministic machine. We have seen how in their various ways the different branches of the new physics have outdated this idea. Quantum physics especially pulls the rug out from under this simple mechanistic image. (p. 235)

Up until rather recently, our own modern science had nothing to say about the plausibility of the mind affecting matter, except that this notion did not fit into its own view of the world, including the classic certainty of Newtonian physics ruling the universe. Within a materialist's model, there simply was no way that thought alone could move matter or that anything supernatural could have an effect on anything natural (assuming that the word *natural* actually means "physical"). If it was true, according to skeptics, that mind powered the physical universe, where was the conduit for such activity? As previously queried, how could something that was not physical in nature *move* something physical? Not until the early part of the twentieth century did heads begin to turn and the pillars of known science begin to collapse, as pillars always eventually do, to reveal a greater truth and understanding (Goswami, Reed, & Goswami, 1993). At this time, in 1927, Heisenberg brought to the world the aforementioned *uncertainty principle.* This newly formulated idea posited that it was not possible to determine with any degree of accuracy the momentum and simultaneous position of quantum particles. Heisenberg stated, "the idea of an objective and real world whose smallest parts exist objectively in the same sense as stones or trees exist, independently of whether or not we observe them, . . . is impossible or at least not entirely possible" (Heisenberg, 1990/1962, p. 83).

Nothing could have upset the Newtonian materialist's applecart more than this. According to Heisenberg, the universe is not a deterministic, massive clockwork ticking away with mathematical accuracy and predictable certainty. He went on to describe this hidden world beneath the known material world as one of *potentia* (Popper, 1958). This term was first used by Aristotle to describe the ethereal world of God's universe. Within the world of potentia all possible events actually exist and reside in a potential form of energy or simply *thought.* These potentials, before becoming manifest particles, do not have a real existence but do have tendencies to exist. In this world of *nothingness*, these potential particles can have contradictory states; in other words, two different positions can be occupied simultaneously. Our own individual observation, or awareness, of a position brings that particle's existence into our conscious material world, and only then is its physical reality presented to us, by choice, or by a belief in its existence.

This potential or tendency, as Heisenberg had described it, was also known as the *wave of possibility*. From this state of nonobserved potential, particles that make up the macro world are pulled, and the corresponding wave of possibility is collapsed to form a physical particle. This collapse is accomplished through observation and is the manner in which our entire three-dimensional world is created. This wave function is then behind every manifest creation of the universe. The wave itself, however, is *passive*; in other words, it cannot collapse on its own and thus needs an agent to bring it into form through observation, awareness, belief, intention, or whatever mechanism of choice is available (Friedman, 1994).

This idea that consciousness collapses the wave of potentiality into material reality opens up the more popular notion, among metaphysicians, that every individual creates his or her own physical reality by collapsing the quantum wave potential into form. What exactly does this mean? Say, for example, there are an infinite number of possible ways you might respond to a situation; all of these ways exist in some state as potential. When you "pick one" of these potentialities, then that quantum wave collapses from a state of "no thing/potential" (wave) to a state of "thing" (particle). The "picking" is the tricky part. Most people believe they do not actually choose much of their reality; it just happens to them. This is where the whole concept of potentia gets dicey. If we bring in eminent physicists John Wheeler's and Hugh Everett's theories positing that all potentia is manifest somewhere in an alternate universe/reality, thus avoiding the collapsing wave idea, understanding the concept can really get messy. Most mainstream quantum physicists do not spend much time contemplating the effects that these theories have on our individual lives; as mentioned before, many do not believe that quantum theory even applies directly to a human being's perception of macro events. Some do, however—Amit Goswami (Goswami, Reed, & Goswami, 1993; Goswami, 2004), David Deutsch (1997; Folger, 2001), and Fred Alan Wolf (1996), to mention a few.

A physicist who might be described as straddling the fence of hard science and metaphysics is David Bohm (1981). Bohm was born in 1917 in Wilkes-Barre, Pennsylvania and pursued an illustrious career as a quantum theorist a bit on the fringe. He taught at Princeton until the Red Scare of the 1950s when he pleaded the 5th Amendment to avoid answering questions presented to him by the House Un-American Activities Committee. He lost his job at Princeton, never to be reinstated. He was, however, acquitted of the charges, but still ended up accepting a professorship far from Princeton at the University of São Paulo in Brazil at the recommendation of Albert Einstein and J. Robert Oppenheimer. Bohm had problems with the Cartesian concept of mind–matter separation and theorized that Heisenberg's wave function consisted of a mass of interconnected energy patterns that make up a realm of reality he termed the *implicate order*. He described this realm as mathematically similar to what is present in a modern-day hologram, at least metaphorically. The patterns in a hologram project an image when light is shone through them in a specified manner. It is interesting to note, as compared with Bohm's implicate order, that the patterns are present in their entirety even if the piece of film in which they were originally interjected is cut into many pieces. Each separate piece is capable of projecting the entire picture. Using the hologram as an analogy, Bohm's universe of unlimited potential is a *whole* system. Every part of it is available to every other part of it simultaneously. Within this structure there is not only an absence of linear time but also no space or distance or dimension of any sort. Every potential simply *is*. "Each portion of space contains information about all portions of space" (Friedman, 1994, p. 54). This sounds curiously familiar and may be a model that could be used to explain the ancient Egyptian concept of reality—a harmonized inner (potential) and outer (physical) reality.

According to Bohm's theory of the implicate order of unlimited possibility, the known or seen world of the explicate order is displayed through an unfoldment of the implicate order. Bohm described this holomovement as containing many levels of wave potential and an infinite number of implicate orders. As these orders unfold, we know them as material reality. What causes unfoldment? Bohm, once again, assigned a term to the causal element in his modality. The operator of the system becomes the *superimplicate order*, which, in effect, causes the unfoldment from the unlimited pool of potential, the implicate order. In his book *Bridging Science and Spirit*, Norman Friedman (1994) explained how Bohm's ideas relate to contemporary quantum mechanics:

> Bohm identifies the quantum field with the implicate order. The superquantum potential he identifies with the superimplicate order, and he goes on to postulate a hierarchy of implicate orders. The second implicate order he calls a source of formative, organizing, and creative activity. The first implicate

> order is engaged in a process of rapid and constant creation and annihilation, which results in an explicate order containing relatively constant, recurrent, and stable aspects of the whole. (p. 70)

All possibility is equally present, and no judgment on quality of existence, such as a desire to determine whether an effect is good or bad, can be logically made. *All* effect exists simultaneously. It is only up to our choice as human beings, in our limited view of *allness*, to experience what we want to experience; as pure consciousness, separate from our physical manifestation, we have an eternity (a *timeless* eternity) to do this. In fact, things *do* matter to us. We are beings who create story and myth and put meaning to life's experiences. As contemporary beings, we also see values, truths, rights and wrongs, and evil and good in the world. I believe this is due primarily to the fact that human beings perceive the universe dualistically in our modern materialist times. We are so far from truly realizing and being aware of our oneness with the universe that we act out of fear and often move further away from this awareness of unity rather than move closer to it. The ancient Egyptians, through their concept of *ma'at* and sacred science, more than likely perceived things quite differently. The innate inner consciousness of the heart that Schwaller de Lubicz describes is the origin of the material outer world. This is the perfect world of *ma'at*, and the creation of the material world was to "do" *ma'at*, to harmonize the outer world of form with the inner world of *ma'at*. The innate knowledge of *ma'at* is the consciousness of the heart.

Bohm's quantum physicist contemporaries did not wholly accept his theories during his lifetime or since, but this is not uncommon among forward-thinking theorists in modern particle physics. Bridging the mysterious gap between the micro and macro world of evident, physical human experience has been difficult, to say the least. Most scientists simply choose to ignore this connection and equally ignore any research or hypothesis that attempts to close the gap. It is then impossible to say that there is any true scientific evidence to support, wholly and unequivocally, the idea that psyche precedes matter in a literal and objective way. However, much conjecture as well as many carefully formulated theories support such an idea.

It is again beyond the scope of this book to discuss in any satisfactory detail the implications that these and many other theories and facts of quantum mechanics have had on the study of consciousness directly, and ancient Egyptian cosmology indirectly, and the suggestion that psyche precedes matter (or thought creates physical form). Certainly, controversy exists behind the broad and sweeping statement that through these quantum discoveries science has finally caught up with what the spiritual sages have been saying for thousands of years. At the very least, however, I believe it is safe to say that quantum mechanics does open the door to more inquiries into the relationship between science and spirituality. It seems that finally modern quantum science (as it has been defined since the inception of the modern scientific method) is saying that there is more to reality than what the Newtonian model has led us to believe for so many years. It may, in fact, be beyond our comprehension to fully understand the nature of reality while we still occupy the physical bodies that, by necessity and for self-preservation, must hold onto certain limited perceptions as truths.

Do we study science to better understand the nature of ourselves as spiritual beings or to better understand the nature of the physical world we observe? Which becomes more important to us as physical expressions on a physical plane of existence? Spirituality and the understanding of our true nature as spiritual beings do not need science as validation. The reverse is true as well: science does not need supernatural underpinnings to make its observation of the world around us valid or useful to our needs as physical entities—at least not science as we have experienced it since the ancient Egyptians' time. This having been said, it is still impossible to separate the two while claiming to understand much of anything at all. We do live and function in a material world, and it is foolish to even hint that science, which now has a remarkable understanding of this world, is useless or even hopelessly confused—it does not, however, present a complete picture.

The question being put forward here is not how ineffective science, as a materialist endeavor, may or may not be, but rather how much *more* effective the perception that the ancient Egyptian concept of *sacred* science would be if put into a current, modern practice. Science, or—more accurately, in this context—materialism, has clearly been operative in bringing humanity a better understanding of the physical world around us and has helped us achieve many miraculous accomplishments. Many of these manifest realizations of modern science, are also indirectly as well as directly responsible for the majority of human suffering as we devise more efficient ways to strip the planet of its natural resources without replenishment, throw the homeostasis of the planet out of kilter, and introduce atomic and chemical pollutants into the atmosphere and environment, which have all but destroyed the natural life-affirming ecology of the planet. This is a description of the global impact of this "half-baked" understanding of reality. On a more personal level, human beings presently live lives filled with a psychic misery that is mired in the muck of dissolution regarding meaning, purpose, and fulfillment. This is certainly not an expression of the consciousness of the heart, where innate natural knowledge is present within each of us to encourage us to "do *ma'at*" and bring harmony, through right action, into our physical reality.

A personal psychology is thus not far behind in expressing its interest in the implications of the observer having a profound effect on material reality. In the collection of her transcribed lectures entitled *Psyche and Matter* (1992), Marie-Louise von Franz, a psychoanalyst and disciple of Carl Jung, presented a variety of arguments and insights regarding the problem of psyche (the inner world of symbols and other imagery) and matter (the outer world of physical manifestation). She investigated how these two worlds respond to one another and how one is integrated with the other. Von Franz cited Jung throughout her lectures and saw his theories on synchronicity and alchemy as the source of the answer regarding this issue. A limitation in von Franz's writing is immediately apparent in this passage:

> However, we do not simply want to regress to the level of primitive magical thought, which believed in a kind of magical causality. Modern science has slowly struggled free of this magical approach only with the greatest of efforts, and it is by no means Jung's intention that we should now fall back into this kind of magical–causal thinking. (p. 22)

It seems that, in the way von Franz attributed to Jung an alignment with modern science, she also was careful not to be quite so unscientific as to give credence to primitive magic as a causal structure (although she did give credence to primitive magic as a synchronistic, acausal structure) (p. 40). She seemed careful to avoid the issue directly by qualifying many of her statements, being certain to differentiate between superstitious thought and meaningful experience. Rational scientific meaning, as opposed to magical meaning, can be found in Jung's theory of synchronicity, which, according to von Franz, seems to be the theory that does unite the inner and outer world. She said:

> When he created the concept of synchronicity, Jung laid a foundation which might lead us to see the complementary realms of psyche and matter as *one* reality. For in each synchronistic event it is the same meaning which manifests in the psyche and also in the arrangement of outer events that occur simultaneously. (p. 40)

Jung saw this acausal connection between an event, say, in a dream, and a matching event in the physical world as being evidence of a relationship between the two that is not dependent on a Newtonian, physical cause and effect. Through Jung's observation and study of synchronicity, a modern window was opened that allowed access to the ancient Egyptian way of experiencing reality, whereby the path between the unseen and nonphysical world and the material world was wide and free flowing.

von Franz (1992) went on to say:

> If we define the collective unconscious as Jung did, as an omnipresent continuum of an unextended presence or an unextended-everywhere, then something that happens at one point, which touches the collective unconscious, has happened everywhere simultaneously. What Jung called an omnipresence he also termed elsewhere a relativity of space-time in the deeper layers of the collective unconscious. This archetypal realm is eternal, i.e., outside time; and also everywhere, i.e., outside space. (p. 161)

This statement is curiously reminiscent of statements found describing the ancient Egyptian concept of space and time, which portray the Egyptian *duat* as beyond time and not bound by the physical restrictions of space. Recall, for instance, Schwaller de Lubicz's (1963/1985) statement regarding the Pharaonic mind:

> [The ancient Egyptian has] faith in an origin that cannot be situated in time and space. This is reality absolute, not to be grasped by our intelligence. This cannot be regarded as a mystery: it is the eternal Present Moment, indivisible Unity. (p. 11)

von Franz (1992) continued to relate these concepts to modern science and thus achieved an integration of ancient esoteric thought, and possibly even magical thought, with modern thinking. While discussing Jung's discovery of synchronicity, she stated:

> This discovery of Jung's—more than many another clue—leads to the postulation that that reality which we seek introspectively to describe as the collective unconscious might be the same unknown and uncognizable reality that atomic physics seeks to describe from the outside as "material" reality. (p. 40)

Quite a bit has been written in the realm of quantum physics about the discoveries of modern theoretical particle science in relation to mysticism and spirituality.

In an interview with von Franz in the documentary film *Matter of Heart* (Whitney & Whitney, 1986), she was asked about her first encounter with Jung when she was 18 years old. She responded:

> He told that story which you can read in the *Memories* about this girl who was on the moon and had to fight a demon, and the black demon got her. And he pretended, or he told it in a way as if she really had *been* on the moon and it had happened. And I was very rationalistically trained from school so I said indignantly, "But she imagined to be on the moon, or she dreamt it, but she wasn't on the moon." And he looked at me earnestly and said, "Yes she was on the moon." I still remember looking over the lake there and thinking, "Either this man is crazy, or I am too stupid to understand what *he* means." And then suddenly it dawned on me, "He means that what happens psychically is the real reality, and this other moon, this stony desert which goes round the earth, that's illusion, or that's only pseudo-reality."

In another segment of the interview, von Franz recalled Jung's visit to his castle at Bollingen after a protracted absence. He had difficulty in the kitchen with the pots and pans—lids clattering to the floor, pots slipping out of hands, and the like. She said he then had a conversation with the pots and pans, apologizing for his long absence and asking them now to cooperate. As a result of his talk, things did settle down. "Everything plays you tricks," she said. "It is naturally your own unconscious mixed up with it. It communicates with matter." von Franz told this story tongue in cheek, but considering what is currently known about Jung and his relationship with the metaphysical and mystical world (especially with the revelations of the *Red Book*, 2009), he may have been more literal in these proclamations than he wished others to think during his lifetime, in which he made great effort to be seen as a serious scientist and medical doctor and not a mystic. A much more detailed discussion on Jung and depth psychology is included in Chapter 7.

It would be remiss not to mention the most obvious demonstrations of the mind–body/psyche-to-matter phenomenon—psi, psychokinesis, mind/body healings, and other aspects of parapsychology. Several of these examples already exemplified could possibly fall under this category—the story of Jung's pots and pans, for instance. Thousands of mystics, sages, shamans, theologians, psychics, and spiritualists, through the ages, have revealed extraordinary gifts and have shown, with varying degrees of reputable evidence, that they can, to varying extents, manipulate or even create matter through means seemingly devoid of a cause-and-effect, physical mechanism. The two considerations, however, in proving or disproving the reality and credibility of these events, are whether they can be measured in a quantifiable way—either through physical evidence or through a consensual, and repeatable, observation of the phenomena—and that they must show no sign of material connection between the person conjuring the event and the event itself; in other words, as in the case of psychokinesis, no hidden wires, magnets, breath, or other physical mechanism can be present to move objects.

Although mainstream science has never fully acknowledged the existence of most of these phenomena, it is difficult to ignore the serious research that has been conducted on behalf of parapsychology and psi, just as it is difficult to dismiss the anecdotal accounts of many supernatural events—as challenging as they may be to prove as factual, they are equally difficult to prove as hoaxes. The more the serious scientific community rejects these phenomena as frivolous tricks and confusions that only the ignorant observer will fall for, the more compelling their defenses become. Mainstream science either ignores or denigrates anecdotal accounts and gives much the same treatment to most of the serious scientific research being conducted in these disciplines such as psi, psychokinesis, the effect of mass consciousness on random number generators, telepathy, remote viewing, reincarnation, and life after death.

The following three paranormal events I present for review are all personal cases of individual people and their encounters with what modern sensibilities would label *supernatural*. Before I begin, a comment on the word *supernatural* is necessary. This term defines a phenomenon as being outside of nature. To be more accurate, I prefer a new term to describe these phenomena—super*material*—which is, in fact, a much more accurate description. Modern science has defined nature as being material, but nature actually should include all phenomena that occur within it, not just physical ones. This is not a new idea, having been pondered by metaphysicians for quite some time.

What do these paranormal events have to do with ancient Egyptian sacred science and modern psychotherapy? The intention in bringing awareness to these cases, and all serious cases that involve the human mind's apparent manipulation of matter, is to present evidence of the human psyche-to-matter issue under discussion here. The paranormal events that include this form of mind manipulation could be considered a very crude and elementary demonstration of mind over matter (obviously not always conscious mind). This concept is relevant here because these cases, if taken seriously, can show us that there is indeed a direct connection between an inner, nonmaterial world and the outer physical world. Needless to say feats of the paranormal are controversial, and it is expected of the reader to carry an open mind as they venture into this intriguing, yet considered by many to be dubious, collection of material.

The first case of the paranormal I will present is the story of Katie, a woman who has experienced the appearance of a thin metal foil that seems to secrete from her pores on her face, arms, and torso. In the late 1980s, Katie's tale was brought to the attention of several researchers and medical doctors and subsequently was presented in an episode of the popular television series *Unsolved Mysteries*. Katie was an illiterate housewife who had no more than a second-grade education and worked as a domestic in Florida. At the time of her investigation, she was in her late 30s and had experienced a variety of paranormal phenomena including sightings of apparitions, materializations of jewelry and gemstones, her own writing of passages in medieval French (she could only write her own name in English and was otherwise illiterate), and premonitions. Using her abilities in this realm, she had assisted the local police force with several cases.

Most of the documentation of Katie's case comes from her psychiatrist Bert Schwarz, who wrote numerous articles about her psychic abilities. Stephen Braude (2007), a professor emeritus of philosophy (and chair of the department) at the University of Maryland, Baltimore County, also witnessed several of Katie's manifestations, which consisted primarily of the aforementioned metal foil material. The substance would form on Katie's face, arms, back, stomach, and legs and appeared to be gold leaf, very thin in nature and bright gold in color. Sometimes, the patches of foil on Katie's body would cover 5 or 6 square inches, at times almost obscuring a third of one side of her face. The results of various laboratory tests on the material proved it to be ordinary brass foil, or commonly called Dutch Metal. Large quantities of the manifested material have been collected and stored over the period of her investigation.

The observation of Katie's materializations were conducted with careful control and attention to being certain she was not carrying the foil concealed on her body or in her clothing. Sometimes, the foil would appear on the investigators or other people present in the room with Katie. It would even appear in closed containers or on other objects, clothes, picture frames, and sealed jars. Although never able to secure a clear video taping of the actual manifestation of the material, the researchers attested to witnessing the foil appearing inexplicably on her skin and her clothing.

Unfortunately, Katie's story ends rather mysteriously. After several years of testing (Katie's materializations were not continuous and would only appear for short periods of time throughout the research period), Katie slipped into obscurity, and her whereabouts are generally unknown.

The second case is that of Ted Serios. Ted was a Chicago bellhop, who discovered sometime in the mid-1960s that he could create images on Polaroid film by merely "thinking" them into existence. Jule Eisenbud (1989), a medical doctor (psychiatry), spent enormous time and effort in relentless research regarding Ted. Hundreds of trials were conducted, resulting in approximately a thousand photographs over a period of about three years. What made Ted's photos unique, compared with any sort of spiritual photography that existed before the invention of instant Polaroid film, was that the results of his efforts were seen immediately, affording no opportunity to fraudulently manipulate the film processing in a lab.

Again, controls implemented in the trials were thorough and stringent, eliminating any possibility that Ted could have been hiding pieces of transparent film that could have been utilized in his images. He simply would project his "thought" into the camera, and the film would be exposed presenting a blurred or strangely affected image, often of buildings or other structures. Some images were pure white, which Eisenbud and Serios called "Whities," whereas others were pure black, called "Blackies." None of these images could have been produced with the normal use of the camera. The pictures are quite compelling, some showing existing scenes of buildings but with odd and unexplainable differences from the actual structures—windows missing or bricked up, parts of buildings missing or radically altered from how they appeared at the time, or images that showed the nature of a structure as it appeared many years before. Some images were difficult or impossible to identify as representations of existing buildings.

The ramifications of this work are astounding, and this brief description does not begin to express the enormity of this research and its implications. Stephen Braude, who also witnessed the Katie manifestations, was present at several later Ted Serios trials.[1] He was also a good friend of Jule Eisenbud and could vouch for his esteemed integrity. One important reason for presenting these two cases out of literally thousands of similar examples of mind-over-matter phenomena is that I have a personal connection with Stephen Braude and thoroughly trust his ability to judge these events as legitimate. He is also a respected member of academia and holds high credentials in his field of philosophy and parapsychology.

The last case, briefly presented, is the story of Ted Owens, also known as the "PK Man." Ted was born in Bedford, Indiana in 1920 to a rather average midwestern family. He was raised by his grandparents, Grandpa and Queenie, who were probably the progenitors of Ted's unique talents due to their own forays into the paranormal with dousing, Ouija board readings, and the like. Ted, later in life, described unusual events as a child, such as several levitations he experienced, all the while being rather uncertain as to what exactly was happening to him. He also had a rather unusual invisible friend, an adult woman who taught him how to read. Ted then became a voracious reader as a young boy, reading everything about aliens, paranormal events, and space travel he could get his hands on.

Ted served in the U.S. Navy during World War I and, after the war, eventually ended up at Duke University in South Carolina at the bidding of J. B. Rhine, the father of experimental parapsychology. Ted became Rhine's assistant, helping him with his writing and research, but, oddly, he never became a star participant in Rhine's laboratory experiments with psychokinesis. It was at Duke, and through his association with Rhine, that Ted became aware that he possessed special psychic skills.

As time passed, Ted became best known for his predictions of weather events—where exactly lightning would strike during a storm, droughts and their end, floods, hurricanes, and the like. His accuracy in these "predictions" (whether precognitive or psychokinetic is difficult to tell) was uncanny, and he became quite famous and popular, as newspapers, magazines, and other news media were anxious to report his successes. Although he did have a few notable "misses," the precision of most of his hits is beyond statistical norms. He claimed to be informed by "Space Intelligences," which he described as extraterrestrial beings who communicated with him through a form of telepathy. He made claims that these "SI," as he called them, would execute his demands and make things happen when he desired them to. Ted had a rather tumultuous career as a skilled "PK Man," always looking for approval and respect and rarely getting what he wanted. He was rather vindictive and often would strike out with punishing blows in the form of disastrous and destructive weather and other events.

Ted's story is relevant, as he seemed to have had control over many macro events such as the major weather disturbances previously noted. If these events were actually created by alien beings, then obviously Ted would possess no superpowers other than telepathy, and his entrance into this narration would be meaningless. To be consistent with the context of this book, I choose to ignore the possibility of an alien connection. (If aliens are responsible for any of this, including the ancient Egyptians' monuments, math, and art, there is, of course, no purpose for this book.)

It is worth investigating Ted's life and activities in more detail, if his story, as it is briefly presented here, is of any intrigue to the reader. Jeffrey Mishlove, a close acquaintance of Ted's and probably the foremost authority on his life and career, wrote the seminal book on Ted, *The PK Man: A True Story of Mind Over Matter* (2000). Again, there are others like Ted, but I chose to include his story because I have a personal association with Mishlove, and I certainly trust his insight and critical acumen.

As extraordinary as these cases may seem to be, there are thousands more just as compelling or even more extraordinary. A multitude of additional cases may not be quite as extreme but still present evidence that is difficult to refute—evidence indicating an innate ability in some humans, and some argue in *all* humans, to manipulate and control matter through only thought or with no apparent material mechanism. Common to most cases, although not all, is the spontaneity of these abilities and manifestations. Most subjects do not seem to have a high degree of control over these skills, and if they do exhibit some control, most often than not, that control is not consistent and reliable.

It is not necessary to believe in the paranormal in order to appreciate the sacred science of the ancient Egyptians. In fact, it is easy to develop an understanding of sacred science devoid of any connection with the paranormal or, more broadly put, the psyche-to-matter process. However, it is easier to contemplate the extraordinary accomplishments, not only in math and astronomy but also in engineering and construction (including the quarry and transport of megalithic stones), if this concept of psyche-to-matter, or mind over body, is at least entertained. I have presented a possible method for mind manipulation of matter, if quantum theory is considered as a viable explanation. Quantum theory has been regarded as the most likely description of how the natural world may present these phenomena (any result we may ascribe to the psyche-to-matter process). It is not the only entertained theory, and it may not be the correct one, but it does present some compelling possibilities.

With this presentation of a few representative modern examples of mind over body or psyche-to-matter phenomena in the form of paranormal manifestations and manipulations, I am not necessarily suggesting that the ancient Egyptians used only their mind to levitate large stones into neat symmetrical patterns in the construction of their pyramids or temples or telepathically guided simple copper tools to cut perfect right angles in solid granite (although these suggestions would not be unreasonable to contemplate). What I am suggesting is that we see ample demonstration in our world today, and in the history of humankind since the ancient Egyptians, of a successful mind-over-body process (if we allow ourselves to believe in the evidence offered). Although most, if not all, of these examples are miniscule compared with the gargantuan feats executed in Egypt, they may all be related to the degree of disciplined control, intention, and belief managed and held by those individuals attempting the executions. Individual psychic abilities and demonstrations are just that—individual. The ancient Egyptian culture consisted of thousands of individuals, all existing within an organized and intentional system with hierarchies of control and doctrine. One can only imagine the potential of that organized mass of individuals, all with singular intention, belief in the rightness of their reality, and dedication to the results of their efforts.

Another important consideration in the psyche-to-matter issue as it may have applied to the ancient Egyptian cosmology is the linear aspect of time. In our modern era, and probably including most of Western thought since the ancient Egyptians, time has been perceived as linear—a movement of experience through a passage including a past, a present, and a future. This linear construct implies time passing, as something has to come before something else. Considering what R. A. Schwaller de Lubicz said regarding the Egyptian concept of time (see quote earlier in this chapter), the ancient Egyptians may not have perceived time in this linear formula of past to present to future.

Continuing this discussion, it is informative to eliminate the human perspective of linear time. Relatively recently modern physics has implied that linear time is actually just a human construct and does not exist unless there is someone around to measure it. In fact, time *is* measurement, not a thing unto itself. Kurt Gödel, considered one of the greatest logicians of our modern era and a close associate of Albert Einstein, suggested that, due to the theoretical possibility of time travel, time itself did not exist; if one can go back to the past, then the past has not in fact passed. Gödel went on to say that time is "a one-dimensional manifold that provides a complete linear ordering of all events in nature" (as cited in Yourgrau,

2005, p. 128). Palle Yourgrau, in his book, *A World Without Time: The Forgotten Legacy of Gödel and Einstein*, quotes Gödel in an explanation of his reasoning:

> This "objective lapse of time" is "directly experienced" and "involves a change in the existing [i.e., in what actually exists]." Time . . . for Gödel, is something "whose essence is that only the present really exists. . . . [It] means (or is equivalent to the fact) that reality consists of an infinity of layers of 'now' which come into existence successively." (p. 128)

If it is true that the linear passage of time as humans perceive it is only an illusion (something that they have conveniently created), then only we, in our limited perception of reality, are capable of putting something in front of something else. If linear time is then an illusion, how does one explain cause and effect as it is related to the psyche-to-matter problem—psyche (thought) being cause, and matter (manifestation of thought) being effect? One explanation is that cause and effect become one and the same; the effect is inextricably intertwined with the cause. In a sense, the effect creates the cause; the need creates the means. Let's review once again Schwaller de Lubicz's (1963/1985) statement about Egyptian time:

> [The ancient Egyptian has] faith in an origin that cannot be situated in time and space. This is reality absolute, not to be grasped by our intelligence. This cannot be regarded as a mystery: it is the eternal Present Moment, indivisible Unity. (p. 11)

The "eternal Present Moment, indivisible Unity"—what can this actually mean other than a "faith" or belief in nonlinear time? Why then might psyche, or thought, or creativity, be required to bring matter, or effect, into manifest reality? If time does not exist, then everything already exists in the present. Everything has already been realized. The cause-and-effect rationale of psyche-to-matter no longer exists; therefore, there is no longer a problem.

Modern humans typically do not fully live in the moment. We do tend to believe that time is linear and that there is a past and a future to contend with as a distinct reality. The ancient Egyptian mind may not have had this perceptual limitation and therefore may have been more adept at allowing the world to effortlessly flow through an eternal present, thus not being limited by the problem of cause and effect. If there is then no first cause (past/present) to create a resultant effect (present/future), there is no need for a conduit to bridge the two together, as there is no "two," no "duality," and no psyche-to-matter "problem."

Note

1 Serios suddenly lost his "powers" in 1967 and never again created images that were clear and discernable, although he did continue to create some amalgamous images and Blackies and Whities.

References

Bohm, D. (1981). *Wholeness and the implicate order*. London, England: Routledge.

Braude, S. E. (2007). *The gold leaf lady and other parapsychological investigations*. Chicago, IL: University of Chicago Press.

Davies, P. C. W., & Gribbin, J. (2007). *The matter myth: Dramatic discoveries that challenge our understanding of physical reality*. New York, NY: Simon.

Deutsch, D. (1997). *The fabric of reality: The science of parallel universes and its implications*. New York: Penguin Books.

Eisenbud, J. (1989). *The world of Ted Serios: "Thoughtographic" studies of an extraordinary mind*. Jefferson, NC: McFarland.

Everett, H., III. (1957). "Relative state" formulation of quantum mechanics. *Reviews of Modern Physics, 29*, 454–462. http://dx.doi.org/10.1103/RevModPhys.29.454

Folger, T. (2001). Quantum shmantum. *Discover, 22*(9), 37–43.

Friedman, N. (1994) *Bridging science and spirit: Common elements in David Bohm's physics, the perennial philosophy and Seth*. St. Louis, MO: Moment Point Press.

Goswami, A. (2004). *The quantum doctor: A quantum physicist explains the healing power of integral medicine*. Charlottesville, VA: Hampton Roads.

Goswami, A., Reed, R. E., & Goswami, M. (1993). *The self-aware universe: How consciousness creates the material world*. New York, NY: Putnam.

Heisenberg, W. (1990). *Physics and Philosophy*. London: Penguin. (Original work published 1962)

Jung, C. G. (2009). *The red book: Liber novus* (S. Shamdasani, Ed.) (S. Shamdasani, M. Kyburz, & J. Peck, Trans.). New York, NY: Norton.

Mishlove, J. (2000). *The PK man: A true story of mind over matter*. Charlottesville, VA: Hampton Roads.

Popper, K. (1958, Summer). The representation of nature in contemporary physics. *Daedalus, 87*, 95–108.

Rosenblum, B., & Kuttner, F. (2011). *Quantum enigma: Physics encounters consciousness*. Oxford, England: Oxford University Press.

Schwaller de Lubicz, R. A. (1985). *The Egyptian miracle: An introduction to the wisdom of the temple* (A. VandenBroeck & G. VandenBroeck, Trans.). New York, NY: Inner Traditions International. (Original work published 1963)

von Franz, M.-L. (1992). *Psyche and matter*. Boston, MA: Shambhala.

Whitney, M. (Director/Producer), & Whitney, M. (Producer). (1986). *Matter of heart* [Motion picture]. USA: Horizon.

Wolf, F. A. (1996). Quantum rules of the universe. In R. E. Dicarlo (Ed.), *Towards a new world view: Conversations at the leading edge* (pp. 58–64). Erie, PA: Epic.

Yourgrau, P. (2005). *A world without time: The forgotten legacy of Gödel and Einstein*. New York, NY: Basic Books.

5

MODERN MATERIALISM AND THE LOSS OF SOUL

The first chapters of this book investigated the majesty and mystery of the products of ancient Egyptian architecture, art, construction, and mathematics. I presented the difficulties in assigning a materialist's paradigm to explain these seemingly magical feats of precision and material manipulation and suggested the possibility that the ancient Egyptians possessed an unusual cosmology that could open up new avenues of execution to explore. For ideas and visions to take physical form in the material world of ancient Egypt would necessitate some method beyond the mechanics and technology Egyptians had at their disposal thousands of years ago. Mainstream Egyptologists seem to believe that these feats were accomplished with nothing more than determination and an abundance of time, using the tools of the period that have been discovered. Further scrutiny, however, has shown this belief to be suspect, at best, and utterly implausible, at worst.

Schwaller de Lubicz, with whom we have become somewhat familiar in these pages, suggested a unique cosmology—a consciousness of the heart, or intelligence of the heart—that could be responsible for a sacred science that the ancients understood and cherished. Sacred science was a pure integration of form and spirit. Consciousness of the heart, driven by a spiritual desire to experience an outer world in harmony with an inner world of sacred knowledge, integrated the seen with the unseen. Various contemporary ideas and examples have been presented that may begin to explain what this sacred science may have been and how it may have been expressed with a psyche-to-matter unfolding. I have also cited examples of the psyche-to-matter process, first with an explanation of the observer effect in quantum mechanics and then with brief descriptions of contemporary instances of paranormal materialization and psychokinesis. These have all been offered simply as ideas and suggestions meant to open the door to further inquiry—but possibly only to questions answered with questions.

This present examination of ancient Egyptian sacred science and consciousness of the heart leads us to our current time and dilemma. What is it about our modern cosmology that keeps from us the knowledge and wisdom of this ancient Egyptian sacred science? Assuming that the ancient Egyptians were indeed human, what did they possess as humans that made them capable of creating what they created with the limited physical means they allegedly possessed? And more importantly, if we do have within us the potential to become conscious of the heart as they did, why can we not access it in a controlled, intentional, and consistent manner? The first primary difference we see in the ancient Egyptian cosmology is their belief that the inner, imaginal, world is real. Mainstream science, upon which most of us rely as the definer of reality, insists that the only real world is the world that is material, measurable, and consensual. The ancient Egyptians experienced this world but also believed that reality included the unseen world, a world that was not measurable or material. These two worlds were of equal importance and possibly were not discernable from one another.

We could refer to the process of bringing this inner world into meaningful relationship with the outer world that our senses perceive as *soul*. The soul of a thing could also be something that is not seen, or detected with the senses (even with the aid of instruments), and not measurable with measuring devices. It then becomes a quality that is sensed without the senses but is simply *known*. For example, we could listen to music or gaze upon art that we feel "has" soul, but are we perceiving soul as an innate quality of the art or music, or is it a process within us that aligns our inner consciousness of the heart, our innate knowledge of the cosmos, with the material world (the music or art) that is stimulating our senses? We could refer to this quality or process with words other than *soul*, but for the purposes of this book, I will stick to the word *soul* to describe it. To clarify soul as we may perceive it today, or as it may be perceived in a more expanded cosmology, I will present several ideas about the history of soul and certain specific definitions of the concept.

Because I am suggesting that something unseen[1] is an integral attribute of something material and seen, I am then placing a meaning on a thing that, according to materialists, is not real (materialists do agree that this unseen attribute may be real in experience, as imagination, but it is not real as in *reality*). In my opinion, and in the opinion of many others, this distinction is the primary fault of a materialist worldview and may be the missing element in our cosmology that made the ancient Egyptians so different and so successful in the execution of a multitude of things in their lives.

Materialism is often considered to be *realism* (although it can be argued that the two terms are not synonymous), a philosophical designation that is defined as a belief that physical objects have an independent existence beyond the act of perception. The opposing doctrine to realism is *idealism*—a belief that nothing exists in physical form beyond what is perceived in the mind. I do not wish to become mired in the details of the philosophies of realism, idealism, panpsychism (all matter is conscious), animism (all matter has a soul), and hylozoism (all matter is inseparable from life). The ancient Egyptians seem to have adhered to some philosophy similar to any, or all, of these last three, but debate rages regarding the nuance and subtlety of these doctrines of reality. What I am trying to convey here is actually much more complex but can be described in a simpler manner. Questioning whether the ancient Egyptians were panpsychics or whether our modern culture is essentially realist is beside the point. What is important here is that the ancient Egyptians adhered to a cosmology that was not solely material and found their reality as an integration of the outer and the inner worlds in such a way that was highly effective in accomplishing the many things they accomplished. They were certainly neither realists nor idealists. As reiterated many times in these pages, I am positing that they saw no distinction, with regard to realness or importance, between the mind and the physical world around them.

This book also does not attempt to present a concise definition of *soul*. Various descriptions are presented here to show the diversity of views regarding what soul might possibly be. None of them is any more accurate than any other, because, ultimately, we do not know what soul actually is; its definition is elusive, and its precise description remains a mystery. This book also makes no claim regarding a distinction between soul and spirit, although some philosophers, theologians, and thinkers have attempted to do so. No attempt is made herein to define soul as emerging from psyche or psyche emerging from soul, as that would imply that linear time is a reality and not merely a human construct (refer to the comments attributed to Gödel in the previous chapter). I am assuming that soul may or may not be separate from consciousness as an autonomous entity that survives without a consciousness to perceive it; in addition, I am not asserting that soul is something to be possessed by an object, although, from a certain perspective, it may certainly appear as if a thing may possess a soul or be animated by one. To describe soul as any of these things assumes a duality or a distinction between soul and the phenomenon to which it is being related. It is, at times, impossible to avoid oversimplification in an objective written work, and possibly the closest one can come in defining soul that would appeal to the dualistic and materialist mindset is through art, poetry, and music. I do suggest, however, that soul is present in all reality, both inner and outer, as the ancient Egyptians seem to have believed, although, in some very significant ways, soul may not be recognized or appreciated. For the purposes of this book, soul can be described in all of the following ways and more, and at the same time, it cannot be described adequately by any of them.

Over the centuries, multitudinous efforts have been made to define *soul* in a variety of perspectives, religious contexts, and literary musings. What seems to be the most uncomplicated in structure is the ancient Greek definition, which presented the word *psyche* as *soul* and defined such as "breath." Philosophers expanded this idea to include life itself, as it could be breathed in and out of a being. Metaphorically, this breathing life can be seen as animation—not necessarily movement that can be seen but rather vibration, which is an attribute of all material things at its most basic level of reduction into ever-moving particles. These definitions still remain within the materialist's realm of physical objects, and for a bit of time in recent history, some believed that the soul of an individual could indeed be measured and even weighed.

Materialist thought has had a corner on the soul market for quite some time. In *The Problem of the Soul*, philosopher Owen Flanagan (2003) contended that *soul*, being the same as mind, is simply another way of describing the physical brain:

> The mind or the soul is the brain. Or better: Consciousness, cognition, and volition are perfectly natural capacities of fully embodied creatures engaged in complex commerce with the natural and social environments. Humans possess no special capacities, no extra ingredients, that could conceivably do the work of the mind, the soul, or free will as traditionally conceived. (p. xii)

This concise statement and viewpoint essentially eradicates any possibility of soul being an attribute that is nonmaterial yet essential in the process of living or, even less likely, active in the process of simply being, as a rock or stone may possess soul—an animistic, or panpsychic, perspective.

The ancient Egyptians defined *soul* in a rather complicated way. Needless to say, they did not believe they were defining the word *soul* as we have truncated it here to one singular concept but instead were merely describing the essence of being. They perceived this essence more as a sort of spiritual development or multiple states of awareness whose description, in the earlier dynasties, was reserved for royalty and the spiritually elite. For them, the essence of the human being existed in three forms: the *ka*, *ba*, and *akh*. The first to consider is the *ka* or, simply put, the vital force behind the living form, which could include human beings, animals, and even plants such as those of crops, which grew infused with the vital energy set within them. For the commoner, this vital energy came forth not from some inner personal psychology but rather from an external force, which bestowed upon the living being the power of life. Upon death, one met with one's *ka*, which was the ancestral force that lay beyond life in the spirit world. In meeting with *ka*, the deceased joined this familial assembly in the spirit world. For the king and for the more spiritually elite, the *ka* was represented as a spiritual double, a doppelganger of sorts, having been created as a sort of parallel representation of the physical being. In some descriptions, this double was physical in form as well, and thus, the true concept of *ka* becomes very difficult to ascertain.

The *ba* is a concept that is often related to the Western perception of soul, although this connection can be misleading as well. In ancient Egypt, the *ba* was encountered only during certain unusual states of consciousness such as those experienced in sleep, initiation, or after-death. The *ba* was also destined for heaven; its purpose was to ascend, and its place was in the heavenly realm, just as the material body was meant to be on earth. The *ba* itself, however, may never have actually reached heaven; instead, *ba* was a term used for the energy of moving toward the spiritual transcendence of heaven. The *ba*, as contrasted with the *ka*, was a more personal representation of the individual and what was left to represent the individual after the death of the body.

The last phase of spiritual transformation in the ancient Egyptians' construct comes in the form of the *akh*. The *akh* is the final stage: complete transcendence into the heavenly realm. Whereas the *ba* was considered still bound to the earth image of the body for certain reasons, the *akh* was deemed completely free of the earth body and, in fact, elicited a new spiritual body known as the *sahu*. This spiritual transcendence was complete, with no earth–body connection, yet still containing some sort of essence of the individual from which the *akh* transcended. This being said, the ancient Egyptians nevertheless had a difficult time perceiving a transformation that in some important way was not associated with the material. They believed that the *ba* was compelled to remain in connection with the decaying body from which it had fled and that the *akh* created the spiritual body, the *sahu*, as a representation of the earthly body. This perception of continuing physicality is difficult to explain and may well be similar to early Western perceptions regarding the images of God and angels and spirits, all still in human form, still dressed in recognizable garb, and still seemingly connected to their earthly physical representation (Naydler, 1996).

Although the Egyptian soul paradigm seems to have only a slight resemblance to the current popular notion of soul, it is noteworthy that the ancient Egyptians created a complex story regarding human spiritual development and evolvement. This belief system was conceived out of the imaginal realm and had no scientific basis (as modern science is defined) that was seated in a materialist reality, although, at all times, the relationship with the physical nature of reality was clearly a defining element. The Egyptian integration of matter and psyche was so thorough and complete that, with our current dualistic way of thinking, we have a difficult time understanding what it meant. Most modern thinkers still describe the Egyptian funerary process, for example, in a limited, literal way, assuming that the Egyptians expected their mummified kings to rise from the dead, eat the food left for them, ride the chariots buried with them, and partake in the physical material objects surrounding their sarcophagi in their permanently sealed tomb buried deep in the earth. With this conclusion, we view the ancient Egyptians as highly superstitious and living an existence departed from reality, when, in fact, they were a highly intelligent and sophisticated culture. It is quite difficult, in our current materialist worldview, to hold two thoughts simultaneously, as the Egyptians more than likely did in their apparent belief that a being could be physical and not physical at the same time, with both realities blended in such a way that there was little or no distinction between the two.

Making a distinction between soul and spirit, James Hillman (1989) suggested that soul still has an earthly connection and is, as a fundamental tenet, dynamically related to the living being with which it is associated, a concept similar to the Egyptian *ba*. He described this place of soul as "a world of imagination, passion, fantasy, reflection, that is neither physical and material on the one hand, nor spiritual and abstract on the other, yet bound to them both" (p. 121). He went on to say that a mistake is made when soul is only seen as a transcendent form of spiritual metaphysics, excluding the experience of suffering and psychological pathology.

This transcendent perspective, indicated Hillman (1989), is left to *spirit*, which he viewed as a more masculine and Apollonian archetype with the quality of perfection and the absolutism of superior truth, similar to the Egyptian *akh*. According to Hillman, soul is imagination, image, moon glow, and the realm of dream and fantasy. Soul can suffer and is vulnerable and soft; it is water as compared with spirit's fire. Whereas spirit knows one unity of truth and is always after ultimates, soul "takes in everything, everything can become soul; and by taking into its imagination any and all events, psychic space grows" (p. 123).

This limited survey of soul is obviously lacking detail. As initially stated, whatever the experience of soul has been throughout human history, it has been described in countless ways, the complexity of which can be staggering, and contradictions in perspective abound. For the purpose of this book, however, a consistent connecting thread is identified through this myriad of views, whereby soul appears as *something else*—an additional something that accompanies a basic state of being: a life, a breath, and an emergent property of the material being-ness of form. Alternatively, does matter emerge from soul? It is impossible to say, and there are arguments regarding soul's primacy to matter and matter's primacy to soul. In a timeless reality, nothing emerges from anything, as all is one, simultaneously; however

> From pharaonic Egypt to Delta blues clubs, from the marble-marveled agora of classical Athens to the vast white tundra of Arctic hunters, belief in an uncanny force at the heart of things has been intuited, a sleepstrange feeling rooted in a *presence* of tremendous impact that circulates through and animates all of nature. (Cousineau, 1994, p. xix)

I have observed that the world of materialistic dogma has not necessarily *lost* soul but has simply ignored it. The value of soul is still respected, for the most part, in the arts, in music, and in other areas of human creativity, where, for die-hard materialists, a bit of the inner world can add flavor and reflective meaning to otherwise mechanical representations of re-formed matter. Soul, however, has seemingly no real conscious or appreciated place in some other important contexts or fields of human endeavor such as medicine, engineering, and most of the applied sciences. The premise of this book suggests that, with modern materialism, the awareness and integration of soul has been lost, or forgotten, or even consciously avoided, which can result in a variety of misalignments in human experience and functionality and may result in a world that appears to have been derailed in its effort to be stable, functional, and harmonious:

> A more familiar litany of descriptions of our fragmented world from any contemporary morning newspaper or evening notebook of a therapist, teacher, or priest would include: a sense of alienation, rootlessness, apathy, burnout, torpor, anxiety, cynicism, the fear of leading an inauthentic life. Every illness has its symptoms, and ours is betrayed by our obsessions, addictions, and

> violence; our corrosive loneliness, vague purposelessness, and hall-of-mirrors narcissism. Soulless times are often marked by black humor reveling in the self-doubt that our lives are mere movie scripts, or, worse, that we're tourists rather than travelers on this road of life. (Cousineau, 1994, p. xxi)

Ancient Egyptian sacred science was a demonstration of *ma'at*, whereby the consciousness of the heart was an intelligence that had at its core an alignment with the intelligence and wisdom of the universe. Through the expression of this alignment, the material world and inner world were in harmony. In this context, and considering the broad definition of soul I have presented here, our present world needs to be more conscious and, specifically, more conscious of the heart in order for this spiritual wisdom to emanate from humankind into the material world that makes up our physical environment. My thesis, as stated before, is that what we call *soul*—again, as it is defined here—becomes the process of blending the inner world, as representation of the perfection of the cosmos, with the material outer world of form. To know soul, to feel soul, to create soul, is to be in tune and in harmony with this innate inner wisdom. It is to walk with God or the gods, to know the divine, and thus to experience it through physical processes. It is to express love, in its most reductionist perspective. This is sacred science. As filmmaker, writer, and lecturer Philip Cousineau (1994) wrote:

> From Socrates, the insatiable seeker after truth, to Ray Charles, the incendiary genius of soul music, the soul-navigating Siberian shamans to Carl Jung in his dream-roving tower at Bollingen, rogue philosophers have observed that the only universe as vast as the one outside is the one inside—one consisting of galaxies of images that have accumulated for billions of years and condensed like stardust in our imaginations. (p. xxii)

To Cousineau's distinguished list of soulful creators I would add the ancient Egyptian priest, pharaoh, and commoner tending their fields of grain in the heat of the life-giving sun, knowing there was more to the wonder of the experience surrounding them than what they saw or felt with their limited physical senses. I describe *soul* here as the catalyst that brings awareness and appreciation for the nonmaterial essence of material things. This nonmaterial essence comes into a human being's awareness through images, dreams, associations, symbols, and stories. It can be understood as an awareness and appreciation of the expanded is-ness of an object, process, or event that takes place in the outer material world.

Moving on to the concept of *materialism*, its definition is self-evident. Its implications, however, are a bit more complicated. To be a materialist, one believes the reality of the material world—in other words, that only things made up of particles that are physical in nature are real. As cited previously, Einstein (1961) had issues with this idea of matter being any longer a viable notion, "since 'matter' has lost its role as a fundamental concept" (p. 161). It has been difficult, however, for materialist science to accept that anything that is not of a physical nature—such as thoughts, dreams, visions, and ideas—is real. Few would deny the fact that we actually do dream and create inner images; however, some argument exists as to exactly what constitutes those images and if, indeed, they have some sort of physical attributes (Rock, 2005).

The concept of materialism possibly began with Democritus's proclamation in the 5th century BCE that all matter is made up of tiny particles called atoms. He put forth the idea that, as matter changes and re-forms into many things, the atoms stay the same, stationary and unchanging (Cartledge, 1999). Two thousand years later, Newton's (1995) *Principia* was published, which reinforced the ancient notion that matter was essentially inert, passive, and made up of all the same material, stacked up and formulated in infinite ways but still essentially reduced to one unchanging element. The universe then came to be viewed as a giant mechanism, with all things and events within it traceable and reducible down to their fundamental reality as tiny, singular *things*.

Astroscientists Paul Davies and John Gribbin (2007) claimed:

> There is no doubt that the Newtonian world view, with its doctrine of materialism and the clockwork Universe, has contributed immensely to the advance of science by providing a highly intuitive framework within which to study a wide range of phenomena. But there is equally no doubt that it has also contributed in large part to alienating human beings from the Universe they inhabit. (p. 13)

How is it, then, that the ancient Egyptians, who did not embrace a doctrine of materialism, could exceed the technological acumen of our modern time with the design and construction of their temples and monuments within the physical limitations of their era? It is assumed that we, in modern civilization, have accomplished all that we have in medicine, architecture, technology, and the sciences in general because we have cast off primitive and superstitious ways and embraced what we believe to be the ultimate truth of the universe—a materialist paradigm. How, then, did the ancient Egyptians, thousands of years before the major discoveries that led us into our current era of scientism and materialism, accomplish so much materially? Their accomplishments are apparent only in what is still tangibly available to us: their temples, monuments, and extant texts. We know little of their internal life, their phenomenology, and how they may have felt living the life they lived, including the meaning, purpose, and fulfillment they may have experienced or gleaned from their existence. We do, however, understand from their extant writings, in particular, the pyramid texts, how they related to death, the gods, and the cosmos.

The beginnings of materialism as the primary tenet of serious modern science sprang forth from a spiritual and religious foundation. Most men and women of science in the 17th and 18th centuries, when science began to be a distinct focus and disciplined activity, were devout theists. In the 17th century, Galileo Galilei, René Descartes, Francis Bacon, Isaac Newton, and Johannes Kepler—who were considered the founders of mechanistic science—were practicing Christians. English statesman and scientist Francis Bacon, sometimes considered the father of the Scientific Revolution, took a quite biblical stance about humans' dominance over nature and essentially claimed his divine right to discover and utilize the mechanistic qualities of the world in which he lived. French philosopher Descartes, who could be considered the founder of mechanistic science, had an early fascination with all things mechanical. In his brief introduction to Descartes' life and thought, philosopher Tom Sorell (2000) noted that Descartes apparently had a vision that the entire universe was made up of infallible mathematical laws, and he did much in his career to create an axiom of science that saw all material existence as mechanical. Sorrell's account clarified that, although a devout Roman Catholic to his dying day, Descartes was often accused of preaching atheistic views, as his theories about a mathematical and mechanistic universe did all but completely do away with God.

The trial of Galileo by the Roman Inquisition in 1633 seems to be the event that finally created the division between science and Christianity. As reported by cellular biologist Rupert Sheldrake (2012), both scientists and theologians agreed to establish separate domains of universal reality—science and religion. Concerns of the heart and soul were left to the Church, and concerns of the mechanics of nature were left to the scientists—at least for the time being. Eventually, observed Sheldrake, the scientists wanted domain over it all, basically eliminating the concerns of the heart and soul as being immaterial and therefore nonexistent. This rise in the influence of science took place in the latter part of the 19th century, when atheism was sweeping Europe, and the basic tenets of an unseen universe under the power of an all-powerful god began to crumble.

Materialism as the foundation of modern 19th and 20th century science received its first major challenges in the early discoveries of physicists such as Werner Heisenberg and Niels Bohr. As explained in the previous chapter, Heisenberg is probably best known for formulating, in 1927, the *uncertainty principle*, which postulates that the position and the momentum of subatomic particles cannot be known simultaneously (Kragh, 1999, p. 207). This discovery led to the postulation of the *observer effect*, which states that a quantum system, when measured, will be affected by the observer measuring it (Rosenblum & Kuttner, 2011, pp. 87–90). Another quantum mechanics discovery that baffled and astounded scientists at the time, including Albert Einstein, was the phenomenon of *action at a distance*, also known as *entanglement* (Rosenblum & Kuttner, 2011, pp. 98, 171). The theory states that if two correlated particles are separated by great distance, and one particle is changed in some way, such as a flip in polarity, the other correlated particle will correspond in the same manner simultaneously—something that could not happen if considering the speed of light. Einstein, even to his death, could not accept what he termed "spooky" action at a distance (as cited in Rosenblum & Kuttner, 2011, p. 7).

These amazing discoveries in the microcosm of physical reality have confounded many, leading to all manner of speculation regarding the definition of what is truly real. Modern physicists, for the most part, ignore the implication of quantum theory's effect on our understanding of consciousness and, instead, concentrate primarily on the mechanics of quantum physics and how knowledge of those mechanics can be used to manipulate the physical world. Others, however, have focused on how quantum physics may shed light on the mechanism that could allow for all manner of things that have hitherto been referred to as *supernatural*.

Parapsychologist and cofounder of the field of transpersonal psychology, Charles Tart (2009), in another exposé on materialism, used the paranormal as evidence against a purely materialistic worldview. In his book *The End of Materialism*, Tart presented a variety of ideas pertaining to spiritualism, materialism, and how modern science is missing a focus on an integral part of humans' reality. The case studies of paranormal phenomena as discussed in Chapter 4 are examples of this possible extension of our presently limited view of reality. As mentioned before, paranormal phenomena are not directly suggested as a spiritual attribute of the ancient Egyptians; these phenomena do fall within the realm of what is considered by materialists to be nonscientific and therefore not real. Parapsychological researcher Dean Radin (1997), in the final chapters of his book, *The Conscious Universe*, made this oddly disturbing comment:

> One possibility is that psi [psychic or paranormal phenomena] will eventually be accepted by the scientific community as little more than a curiosity, a psychological reflection of the quantum interconnectedness of the universe. Possibly it will go no further than that. (p. 288)

Radin, like Tart and Sheldrake, seemed to imply that a scientific and materialist acceptance of any sort is the primary goal of psi research. It also seems, to a large degree, that the goal of many studies on spirituality and science are attempting to bring spirituality to an understanding through materialist science and not the other way around. Although all of these studies are useful to pave the way toward an understanding of the ancient Egyptian concept of sacred science, it is crucial to understand that a scientific, material cosmology will not sufficiently explain the process of soul or, in Schwaller de Lubicz's terms, the consciousness of the heart.

Ken Wilber (2001b), an influential and widely read American philosopher, edited an anthology entitled *Quantum Questions: Mystical Writings of the World's Greatest Physicists*. With this collection of essays, Wilber presented the views of prominent figures in quantum physics as gleaned from their own personal knowledge. In his preface to the book, Wilber (2001a) warned his readers that "modern physics offers no positive support (let alone proof) for a mystical worldview" (p. xi) but added, "Nevertheless, every one of the physicists in this volume was a mystic" (p. xi). Reading their intimate accounts is enlightening and does help to improve understanding of the implications of quantum theory and how this unusual science relates to religion and ancient teaching. The material paradigm to which most scientific research adheres begins to become a bit murky at the quantum level. This fact is probably why so many scholars and students of mysticism and spirituality turn to quantum science when looking for the bridge that may connect science and spirituality; turning in this direction may, at least, begin to explain some of the ancient teachings and how those teachings may have a scientific basis. It is difficult to say whether this attempt to legitimize spiritual knowledge with science is truly relevant to bringing a deeper spiritual practice, and thus a sense of soul, back into the materialistic foundation in which most of the world and its inhabitants seem to be immersed.

In continuing our discussion regarding bringing the inner, spiritual world up to importance and prevalence equal to that granted to the physical, material world, we face a formidable hurdle in modern science's insistence that only what is material and measurable is real, and all else is merely illusion. Rupert Sheldrake has spent much of his professional life attempting to expand modern science's view of the natural world to include phenomena outside of its own dogmatic and presumptuous doctrines. In his most current book, *Science Set Free*, Sheldrake (2012) discussed the ten most prominent dogmas of science, which include these questions, along with six others: "Is Nature Mechanical?" "Is Matter Unconscious?" "Is Nature Purposeless?" and "Are Psychic Phenomena Illusory?" In answering these ten questions about assumptive modern science, Sheldrake presented ideas as well as evidence that illustrate a conventional, materialist, blindness that obscures the whole truth about reality.

Sheldrake (2009) presented his ideas about morphogenetic fields in his book *Morphic Resonance*. The concept of morphic resonance, as Sheldrake discussed it, could very well be the explanation for much that has been experienced in paranormal and spiritual realms. Morphic resonance could also be an explanation for Jung's concept of archetypes and the collective unconscious. According to Sheldrake (1987):

> Jung thought of the collective unconscious as a collective memory, the collective memory of humanity. He thought that people would be more tuned into members of their own family and race and social and cultural group, but that nevertheless there would be a background resonance from all humanity: a pooled or averaged experience of basic things that all people experience (e.g., maternal behavior and various social patterns and structures of experience and thought). It would not be a memory from particular persons in the past so much as an average of the basic forms of memory structures; these are the archetypes. Jung's notion of the collective unconscious makes extremely good sense in the context of the general approach that I am putting forward. Morphic resonance theory would lead to a radical reaffirmation of Jung's concept of the collective unconscious. (p. 25)

Most mainstream scientists do not readily accept Sheldrake's ideas, and he remains on the fringes of materialist thought; however, Sheldrake considers himself a serious scientist (much like Jung thought of himself), believing in the current model of the scientific method of experimentation and empirical experience to prove his theories. He has made great effort to apply this method, and many of his hypotheses are backed by empirical evidence that he has gathered through carefully constructed, scientifically robust experiments.

Sheldrake believed that fields, much like magnetic fields, devoid of any material elements, are responsible for much that is experienced that has been labeled *supernatural* or *paranormal*. He found these fields responsible for any psi phenomena such as telepathy and telekinesis as well as for much that a more material, scientific explanation has previously attributed to the function of genes, DNA, and certain behavioral and psychological phenomena such as the process of learning (2012, pp. 231–259). Sheldrake believed that the limited number of genes in genetic coding is insufficient to explain the huge diversity in human cellular development and human characteristics (pp. 168–171). He purported that memory is a result of morphogenetic fields and cited the current trace theory of memory (whereby memory is deemed dependent on a substance that resides in the brain) as unsupported by any substantial evidence (pp. 187–211).

More important, however, is whether or not Sheldrake's theories indicate the limitations of materialist science. Science makes many claims about the reality of the world; most of them, according to Sheldrake, are not provable through normal scientific methods and are therefore just assumptions. The idea that stands at the forefront of these dogmas is that only what is made of physical matter is real. Sheldrake claimed that this dogma alone has stopped most people from paying serious attention to their unseen nature and the unseen and thus unscientific nature of the world around them. The subjective and inner imaginal world then remains relatively unimportant in today's Western culture, as it has never received the serious regard that the material world is given and therefore does not have a powerful or authoritative voice in people's overall experience of life.

A respected scientist who possibly agreed with Sheldrake's theories was quantum physicist David Bohm, whom we have already met in Chapter 4. Recall Bohm's (1981) postulation that the universe is made up of what he labeled *implicate* and *explicate order*. The implicate order is the realm of potentiality and possibility, and the explicate order is formed by an unfoldment of the implicate order—this is the material world that humans see and within which they function physically. Bohm often used the concept of holography as an analogy to his theory, stating that the whole of the universe is present within the smallest of its parts. Because the implicate order exists outside time and space and is made up of infinite possibility, it has no quantifiable attributes—again, much like the ancient Egyptians described their Far-World, a place outside of time (Baigent, 2006, p. 160).

Michael Talbot (1991) investigated the discoveries of Bohm in depth and explained how they shed light on ancient as well as modern spirituality. In his book *The Holographic Universe*, Talbot discussed a variety of topics relating to the concept of an interconnected universe—a universe of unity and wholeness. He related Jung's ideas about the collective unconscious and universal archetypes to Bohm's concept of implicate and explicate order and emphasized the existence of an interconnecting field or web that connects all things and relates all things to each other (pp. 60–61). Although Talbot did not mention Sheldrake's morphogenetic field theory in particular, many of the concepts discussed, most notably Bohm's model of reality, are similar in nature and function.

Sheldrake's concept of morphogenetic fields and Bohm's views on implicate and explicate order are essentially antimaterialist concepts, presenting an obviously nonmaterial explanation for much of what is called *reality* as well as bringing into the definition of natural phenomena much that has been deemed supernatural, such as psychokinesis, telepathy, and other anomalous experience. Although not typically recognized as soul, these unseen fields of effect could be understood as the missing soul of materialism—or at least the carriers of the essence of soul. They may be essentially functional in a material environment, such as the way a gravitational field is functional as it relates to its material environment; these fields could be the conveyance of information that defines soul, or that functions as soul, but not soul itself.

In another essential text by Talbot (1992), *Mysticism and the New Physics*, the author stated, "For centuries the mystic has asserted that matter and consciousness are different aspects of the same *something*" (p. 30). He then implied that the new physics (quantum physics) has a message for everyone that indicates that human beings are active participants "in a universe of ever-increasing wonder" (p. 30). He added that "we have penetrated matter and found a bit of maya—and a glimpse of ourselves" (p. 30). In his text, Talbot also related a story from the infamous don Juan tales of Carlos Castaneda. In *Journey to Ixtlan*, both Castaneda (1972) and his mentor, don Juan, are in the desert at night searching for a spirit. They come across what Castaneda observed to be a calf-like creature with the ears of a wolf and the beak of a bird. It is curled up in their path and screaming as if about to die. Castaneda, at his first encounter with this beast, is terrified; but soon, after his reasoning powers kick in and assure him that the existence of such a creature is impossible, he sees that it is actually a fallen tree branch wafting about in the wind. He points this out to the Yaqui shaman and expresses his pride in seeing the *true* reality. Don Juan rebukes him and tells him that in fact the tree branch *was* a dying spirit while it was "alive with power" (p. 104) and that it was not transformed into a tree branch until Castaneda doubted its existence. Talbot (1992) commented:

> If we believe that an "out there" reality exists, we are probably inclined to react like Castaneda. We arrange the world until we once again perceive our one cherished Environment. . . . But we should be cautious and not pass judgment on its realness. It is most assuredly like Schrödinger's cat. Its reality and its unreality are solely contingent upon how the collective arranges the world. (p. 96)

Talbot's reference to Schrödinger's cat is an allusion to the famous quantum physicist's thought experiment that suggested that two opposing states of reality could exist simultaneously.

B. Alan Wallace, a researcher who explores the intersection of consciousness studies and scientific disciplines, presented an argument regarding science's narrow view of reality and, much like Sheldrake's (2012) argument in *Science Set Free*, Wallace (2000) made significant points regarding science's dogmatic approach to the nature of reality and what he called *scientific materialism* (pp. 21–39). One such point is the following:

> While scientific materialism actually subsumes science and scientific realism, it is often misleadingly equated with science itself, especially by its advocates. Although the claims of scientific materialism go far beyond the legitimate domains of science, most scientific research is now conducted within the metaphysical framework of this ideology. Thus, it is easy to conflate the two, but in so doing, one overlooks possibilities for scientific research that do not conform to this belief system. (p. 21)

Wallace's argument is similar to Sheldrake's assertion that what is narrow-minded and dogmatic is not science itself but rather scientists' resistance to change and refusal to look beyond the assumptions of modern scientific perspectives. Although this book's presentation of ancient Egyptian sacred science as the basis for a new modality of psychotherapy is not directly concerned with the scientific validity (as defined by modern science) of ancient Egyptian cosmology, it is concerned with the loss of soul in modern materialism and the presence of soul in the ancient Egyptian sacred science. Wallace pointed out, as Sheldrake and others do, that current scientism is limited both in its own definition of reality and in the practice of its methods.

In his book *Relativity: The Special and the General Theory*, theoretical physicist Albert Einstein (1961) had the following to say about this issue of materialism and the loss of the inner world perspective:

> All these space-like concepts [meaning objective space, time, matter] already belong to pre-scientific thought, along with concepts like pain, goal, purpose, etc. from the field of psychology. Now it is characteristic of thought in physics, as of thought in natural science generally, that it endeavors in principle to make do with "space-like" concepts alone, and strives to express with their aid all relations having the form of laws. The physicist seeks to reduce colours and tones to vibrations, the physiologist thought and pain to nerve processes, in such a way that the psychical element as such is eliminated from the causal nexus of existence, and thus nowhere occurs as an independent link in the causal associations. It is no doubt this attitude, which considers the comprehension of all relations by the exclusive use of only "space-like" concepts as being possible in principle, that is at the present time understood by the term "materialism" (since "matter" has lost its role as a fundamental concept). (p. 162)

Granted, before science and the scientific method came to be regarded as the arbiter of truth and reality in our Western-dominated world culture, religiosity and superstition ruled the masses in most parts of the Western world (Hamilton, 2003; Michelet & Allinson, 1992). The influence that Judaism, Christianity, and Islam had on this monotheistic paradigm is beyond the scope of this book to explore. Suffice it to say that much of the Western world was under the power of a religious dogmatic organization that molded the more metaphysical, ineffable, and mystical tenets of ancient wisdom traditions into a predominantly ruthless, patriarchal ruling system (Picknett, 2003; Picknett & Prince, 2011). Notable exceptions were the mystics in all the major religions, who were quite active during this period and practiced a much broader interpretation of sacred texts and concepts. Great accomplishments were made in the name of Christianity, Islam, and Judaism, including, from a materialist's perspective, the many splendid cathedrals and mosques built throughout the world, advances in medicine, engineering, and astronomy to name a few. Luminaries such as Meister Eckhart, Thomas Aquinas, Moses Cordovero, and Jalāl ad-Dīn Muhammad Rūmī stood out from the crowd and brought to the world imaginative and soulful insights from the ancient religious texts of their disciplines as well as general interpretations of life and the nature of God. All too often, however, these men and women were persecuted and frequently put to death for views that were considered heretical (Furlong, 1996, pp. 5–7; Harmless, 2008, p. 83; Matt, 1995, pp. 13–15; Woods, 2011, p. 5).

In his book, *The Taboo of Subjectivity*, B. Alan Wallace (2000) wrote, "Scientific materialism has obscured the subjective world pertaining to the nature, origins, and function of the mind and consciousness and has obscured the relation between the inner world of consciousness and the outer world of the objects of consciousness" (p. 56). This statement can be seen as an argument for a more sacred science as contrasted with a more materialist science. In the circles of scientific endeavor (with some notable exceptions such as Einstein, as previously cited), whose possibly naïve intention is the pursuit of truth, it has been assumed that science must be limited to the Newtonian laws of the universe—a materialistic set of laws. It may be time, as Wallace implied, for science to be expanded to include the sacred, the holy, and the soul inherent in the inner world of consciousness. Still, to many, the idea of returning to a more mystical, inner orientation or even allowing that inner world an equal say in their operating structure is tantamount to returning to the dark ages of superstition and irrational, destructive behavior. At the same time, it does not seem fair to compare the larger, more fully integrated, sacred world paradigm of the ancient Egyptians and other pre-Christian era cultures with the two-dimensional views of post-Christian Western life. This predominately negative view, however, seems to be one of the major arguments in favor of scientism and materialism and against allowing equal consideration to the inner, imaginal world.

Today, indisputably, we live in a world where materialist science has provided inestimable wonders. Medicine has advanced to a state that has reduced much of life's physical suffering and certainly has been instrumental in increasing our physical comfort and our life expectancy. Our physical knowledge of the universe and the rest of the natural world in which we engage as well as the technological wonders science has brought us are clearly advantageous in many regards. All of this is available to us as a result of our materialist paradigm, or so it seems. The awareness of soul, or utilization of it, still often manages to creep in where it is not altogether welcome, albeit probably less and less as the years wear on. In terms of oversimplification of the issues at hand, it is important as well not to conflate science with materialism. A scientific materialism certainly exists, but science does not necessarily have the intention to limit itself to material investigation alone (although its dictionary definition certainly implies that). The romantic pursuit of science, in its beginning, was to learn of the mind of God through his creation, which does not necessarily imply a strictly materialist approach. As the pursuit of science ensued, however, these early scientists began to find it increasingly difficult to see a nonmaterial God as the purveyor of all that is in material existence.

The ancient Egyptians also saw science as sacred in all of their physical endeavors, architecture, medicine, art, temple construction, and military campaigns and, presumably, in their every day social life. I believe that in modern times as well, a sacred or soul-aware way of living[2] could benefit just about all facets of engagement in our physical lives.[3] The architect, the doctor, the artist, the engineer, the scientist, the accountant, the mother, the student, the child at play, and all others can benefit by bringing more soul awareness into their lives.

Throughout this book, I make the broad suggestion that modern materialism has lost soul (or is actively ignoring it), implying that following the ancient Egyptian way of sacred science will bring back the soul that humanity desperately needs. This statement, of course, is not altogether accurate. As with most anything, the truth is not that black and white. Relevant to this statement, I also hold to the belief that soul is always present, and reclaiming it is simply a matter of recognizing it and inviting it into consciousness—or, if soul is indeed a process of becoming aware of the consciousness of the heart, to allow a facilitation of that process. As repeated throughout this text, the loss of soul in modern materialism is viewed as the result of the seemingly conscious choice to demote the inner world to a place of mere curiosity (if even that) rather than to a place of meaning, integral purpose, and equality with the outer, material world. It appears to be commonplace that we, as individuals as well as generally as a culture, tend to view any meaning we might find in this inner world to be superstitious and ultimately useless. At best, it may be entertaining and curious and, at worst, dangerously influential—such as the decision to postpone what is presented as a life-saving surgery, due to a dream or other intuitive insight. This inner world appears in our current modern culture as a peculiarity, an abstraction of sorts, which resides within what we perceive as our rational, objective, reality. Dreams, imagination, gods and goddesses, archetypal symbols, rituals, intuition, and even paranormal events such as extrasensory perception (ESP), psi experiences,[4] ghosts, spirits, and the like all fall into a category of possible interest but of an ultimately useless variety. Only in art or possibly psychology are these inner events taken to be useful or vitally revealing, but they still are typically not regarded as *real* in and of themselves, in the sense of being essential and with purpose and meaning equal to things that occur in a material form.

The problems of materialism drew my attention and called me to write this book. I have a profound interest in modern materialistic science, particularly medical science, for the reason that it deals directly with the human organism and its conflict with soul awareness and the inner world, where all experience, all material manifestation, and, thus, all of nature is integrated into a wholeness of being. I have chosen the sacred science of ancient Egypt above all other similar cultures as a conduit or trajectory into the current problem of the loss of soul in modern materialism primarily because of a general awareness of the lack of the inner, imaginal world, in materialist science. Ancient Egyptians were known specifically for their amazing material feats in architecture, medical science, and crafts. In my view, it is remiss to assume that all these objective achievements were carried out based solely on a modern materialistic perspective. Evidence has shown this assumption to be wildly inaccurate.

My personal interest in modern materialism, reductionist science, and the seeming lack of soul in our current Western culture is difficult to extract from my metaphysical interests, parapsychological interests, and, obviously, my interest in Egyptian sacred science. Having experienced the death of my first wife from cancer in 2003 and the objective and scientific modern medical process she encountered through her brief illness, I was left utterly confused and bewildered concerning how such a soul-filled experience—the illness and subsequent death of my wife—could be handled by many of her healers and caregivers (the medical machine) in such a cold and soulless manner. At first, I attributed this concept of lost soul only to the medical establishment, as that was my focus at the time. Myron Denney (2001), a medical doctor turned depth psychologist, commented on this difficult situation in the medical field:

> The modern medical healing arts are caught in the prevailing scientific paradigm of Western culture, functioning with a biomedical science that privileges quantity over quality, fragmentation over wholeness, and matter over spirit. As a result, the emotional, spiritual, and soulful aspects of healing are often neglected. (p. iii)

The medical field seems to be the most obvious area in our contemporary culture that would benefit from a return to the awareness of soul, but it is not the only one by far.

In our modern materialist culture, we typically see no value in the injection of soul into our sciences, finding this best left to art and other forms of subjective expression. Very few will see a value in a medical doctor singing a song, reciting poetry, or playing the harmonica before a surgery or even disclosing with the surgical team a personal accounting of the patient on whom they are about to operate (Denney, 2012). When my wife, Janice, was ill and struggling with her long downward slide in health due to cancer and its subsequent chemical treatment, I personally experienced, again and again, an awareness of soul in an otherwise cold, objective, medical paradigm of care. On one occasion, one of her primary doctors, Mike DelaTorre, helped Janice to the car from the Block Medical Center in Chicago after a particularly difficult day of chemotherapy. I discussed this occasion in the following excerpt from a book I authored after Janice's death, written from the perspective of writing a letter to my wife Janice:

> Mike wheeled you out in your wheelchair to the car. It was bitter cold and dark with cloud cover and approaching evening. The Chicago sky was spitting a few snowflakes here and there. Mike helped you out of the wheelchair into the car. I looked at Mike's face and was struck by the sincere care and compassion I saw there. "Thank God for these people," I thought. It was unfathomable to me to think of this journey alone. Our needs transcended mere objective health care, as do anyone's needs when faced with this sort of formidable health challenge. I had gotten to a point where I truly didn't care anymore about the medical technology. It seemed we had exhausted those possibilities long ago. I thought of the line from the movie *AI* that had struck a chord with me: "This situation is beyond our science." Yes, Janice, I began to feel that our situation was indeed beyond our science. The science no longer seemed to matter. What did matter was love, compassion, and sincere empathy—intention to care.
>
> It seemed so long ago that I had posed my "difficult" question to all of your doctors—"Is it your intention to cure Janice?" Was it Mike's intention to cure you as he so lovingly took you out to the car that snowy evening? I doubt it. But it did seem it was Mike's intention to love you and to care for you as best he knew how. You were beyond his science, but you were not beyond his human and divine ability to care. This was true for all of "your people" at Block. They were angels. (Hayen, 2003, p. 212)

Janice's doctor's behavior was not bedside manner per se, as bedside manner can be taught objectively, and if the science of medicine shows a bedside manner has positive efficacy, it can then be integrated, objectively, into the standard of care to which licensed physicians adhere. This experience illustrates something quite different. Dr. DelaTorre's treatment comes from the heart, not the head, and is an inner world connection that is largely ignored by medicine at best, and even discouraged at worst. Here is soul made manifest through care and love, but it is also an awareness of a suffering soul that touches the wounded heart through empathy and understanding. The soul present here in this experience is the soul described by James Hillman, which follows and absorbs the life experiences and expansions of awareness and consciousness through suffering and illness.

The Egyptians' paradigm of sacred science, along with the presence of soul or utilization of the process that soul elicits, integrated throughout their entire experience, both internally and externally, and their seamless incorporation and acceptance of the divine, sacred, and imaginal into their worldview, is a perspective that I believe would enrich our current paradigm of scientism and materialism. Common sense would dictate, in most situations, that it would be a mistake to return to the specific rituals and general ways of the ancients; instead, it might be beneficial to apply our knowledge and understanding of the ancient Egyptian spiritual paradigm to our own modern sensibilities, as best we are able to do.

I close this chapter with the poignant words of Jeremy Naydler (2009) as he described the ancient Egyptians:

> This was a culture for which the world was still permeable, into which a spiritual light shone, illuminating it with a divine radiance. The gods were still present in the land of Egypt, for nature was still transparent, not yet solid and opaque. Nature mediated divine energies that people became aware of by "seeing through" the phenomenal world to the numinous presences beyond. (p. 90)

Notes

1 Using the words "unseen" and "seen" can be rather confusing. I am not referring to "seeing" with eyes, but rather using the word to denote the material, physical, world. The "unseen" world, which is referred to here as well, is meant to denote not a world too small, too far away, or too large, to be seen with eyes, but rather the nonmaterial, nonphysical world.
2 Please note that I am not specifying a *religious* or even *spiritual* way of living.
3 The word *physical* is used here also to denote humanity's spiritual activities, as we, in our living form, are still functioning and engaging with a *physical* world.
4 *Psi*, a letter in the Greek alphabet and first letter of the word *psyche*, "is the term parapsychologists use to generically refer to all kinds of psychic phenomena, experiences, or events that seem to be related to the psyche, or mind, and which cannot be explained by established physical principles" (Varvoglis, 2009, para. 1).

References

Baigent, M. (2006). *The Jesus papers: Exposing the greatest cover-up in history*. San Francisco, CA: HarperSan Francisco.

Bohm, D. (1981). *Wholeness and the implicate order*. London, England: Routledge.

Cartledge, P. (1999). *Democritus*. New York, NY: Routledge.

Castaneda, C. (1972). *Journey to Ixtlan: The lessons of don Juan*. New York, NY: Simon.

Cousineau, P. (1994). *Soul: An archaeology—Readings from Socrates to Ray Charles*. San Francisco, CA: HarperSanFrancisco.

Davies, P. C. W., & Gribbin, J. (2007). *The matter myth: Dramatic discoveries that challenge our understanding of physical reality*. New York, NY: Simon.

Denney, M. (2001). *Body, soul, and medicine: Confessions of an elder physician* (Doctoral dissertation). Available from Proquest Dissertations and Theses database. (UMI No. 3029756)

Denney, M. (2012). *Nobody's boy: An old doctor and a new science* [Kindle DX version]. Retrieved from http://www.amazon.com/Nobodys-Boy-Doctor-Science-ebook

Einstein, A. (1961). *Relativity: The special and the general theory; A popular exposition*. New York, NY: Crown.

Flanagan, O. J. (2003). *The problem of the soul: Two visions of mind and how to reconcile them*. New York, NY: Basic Books.

Furlong, M. (1996). *Visions and longings: Medieval women mystics*. Boston, MA: Shambhala.

Hamilton, B. (2003). *Religion in the medieval West* (2nd ed.). New York, NY: Oxford University Press.

Harmless, W. (2008). *Mystics*. New York, NY: Oxford University Press.
Hayen, T. M. (2003). On the very edge of magnificence. Unpublished manuscript.
Hillman, J. (1989). *A blue fire: Selected writings* (T. Moore, Ed.). New York, NY: Harper.
Kragh, H. (1999). *Quantum generations: A history of physics in the twentieth century*. Princeton, NJ: Princeton University Press.
Matt, D. C. (1995). *The essential Kabbalah: The heart of Jewish mysticism*. San Francisco, CA: HarperSanFrancisco.
Michelet, J., & Allinson, A. R. (1992). *Satanism and witchcraft: The classic study of medieval superstition*. New York, NY: Carol.
Naydler, J. (1996). *Temple of the cosmos: The ancient Egyptian experience of the sacred*. Rochester, VT: Inner Traditions.
Naydler, J. (2009). *The future of the ancient world: Essays on the history of consciousness*. Rochester, VT: Inner Traditions.
Newton, I. (1995). *The principia*. Amherst, NY: Prometheus Books.
Picknett, L. (2003). *Mary Magdalene: Christianity's hidden goddess*. London, England: Robinson.
Picknett, L., & Prince, C. (2011). *The forbidden universe*. London, England: Constable.
Radin, D. I. (1997). *The conscious universe: The scientific truth of psychic phenomena*. New York, NY: HarperEdge.
Rock, A. (2005). *The mind at night: The new science of how and why we dream*. New York, NY: Basic Books.
Rosenblum, B., & Kuttner, F. (2011). *Quantum enigma: Physics encounters consciousness*. Oxford, England: Oxford University Press.
Sheldrake, R. (1987). Part I: Mind, memory, and archetype: Morphic resonance and the collective unconscious. *Psychological Perspectives, 18*(1), 19–25.
Sheldrake, R. (2009). *Morphic resonance: The nature of formative causation*. Rochester, VT: Park Street Press.
Sheldrake, R. (2012). *Science set free: 10 paths to new discovery*. New York, NY: Chopra Books
Sorell, T. (2000). *Descartes: A very short introduction*. New York, NY: Oxford University Press.
Tart, C. T. (2009). *The end of materialism: How evidence of the paranormal is bringing science and spirit together*. Oakland, CA: Noetic Books/New Harbinger.
Talbot, M. (1991). *The holographic universe*. New York, NY: HarperCollins.
Talbot, M. (1992). *Mysticism and the new physics*. London, England: Arkana.
Varvoglis, M. (2009). What is psi? What isn't? Retrieved from http://archived.parapsych.org/what_is_psi_varvoglis.htm
Wallace, B. A. (2000). *The taboo of subjectivity: Toward a new science of consciousness*. New York, NY: Oxford University Press.
Wilber, K. (2001a). Preface. In K. Wilber (Ed.), *Quantum questions: Mystical writings of the world's great physicists* (pp. xi–xii). Boston, MA: Shambhala.
Wilber, K. (Ed.). (2001b). *Quantum questions: Mystical writings of the world's great physicists*. Boston, MA: Shambhala.
Woods, R. (2011). *Meister Eckhart: Master of mystics*. London, England: Continuum.

6

CONTEMPORARY PIONEERS OF THE NEW SACRED SCIENCE

In our modern time we may have to see sacred science as a process rather than as a paradigm or concept that the ancient Egyptians took for granted within their cosmology. A process, because the task at hand is for our culture to begin to see what the ancient Egyptians saw without effort: a material world and method of creation that was infused with spirit and spirits, where what we would now call *soul* was expressing. According to the ancient Egyptians, this resulted in *ma'at*, a harmony between the inner and outer world. This concept should be quite clear to the reader by now, as it has been repeated in various ways throughout this book.

We are now faced with the question: *How do we implement this process of sacred science?* In other words, how do we perceive our material world as infused with spirit and spirits and reawaken an awareness of soul in all things or soulfully create within us an awareness or consciousness of the heart and all that that consciousness entails—a harmonious inner and outer world. Schwaller de Lubicz said, "We must be able to transcribe what is in us into our mental and objective consciousness, by establishing a relationship between the life in us and observation of that life in Nature" (1960/1985, p. 14). Has anyone since the ancient Egyptians attempted to engage in this process? I believe the answer to that question is a resounding yes. As human beings, we certainly often feel an alignment with an inner truth. Through a practice of spirituality this is probably indeed quite prevalent. Through the expression of art, music, or literature as a creator, an interpreter, or observer, we become aware of something divine, otherworldly, and deeply resonant within us—as we do when engaged with nature, experiencing a sunset, or looking into the eyes of a loved one. I believe this is an awakening of the consciousness of the heart, an alignment with a universal intelligence and order. Some, needless to say, would call this the work of God; others would say it was the evidence of soul or a recognition of soul.

Must we limit the physical events that bring about this numinous experience? Can we be moved spiritually by an accountant's ledger sheet, the chemical reaction in a person's body from a pharmaceutical intervention, or the mathematical precision required to build a suspension bridge? Or can we see spirit in even (seemingly) less miraculous experiences—the manner in which the bright rays of the morning sun cut across a kitchen table, the smooth feel of cold granite under our hand, or the (seemingly) uneventful life of a river stone sitting on a bedroom shelf? What is divine?—the spectacular? What is spectacular? Worship everything that you see and sense—*every thing*. This is the *process* of sacred science.

Medicine is often criticized for its lack of soul, or heart, but at the same time, the practice of medicine is expected to have its foundation solidly in material, objective, and quantifiable science. It would be difficult to imagine, in our modern times, a thorough integration of science and heart in medical practice without the fear of superstition creeping in—and how would our modern sensibilities define allowing a physician's dream world or imagination to influence his or her medical decisions other than as superstition? From this present perspective, the process of sacred science becomes an integration of *conscious* science and *conscious* heart or soul. It would seem imperative that an awareness and acceptance of the value and worth of the unseen forces of the heart and soul be present—at least for this holistic approach to be most effective. This would be a difficult proposition within our current worldview. This awareness, or process, of soul awareness would have to be approached delicately and in quite small doses to be acceptable. I do believe we are experiencing this awareness in our current time, albeit very subtly, and possibly for the wrong reasons (being still within a materialist context).

As pointed out in previous chapters, we may see an abundance of expression of a consciousness of the heart in our modern time, but typically only in areas that materialist science has not permeated to such a deep level, such as spirituality, art, and literature. Medicine, physics (macro physics), and any or all of the hard sciences as well as government, economics, ecology, agriculture, education, and certainly mental health are in dire need of more conscious soul awareness, thus creating a *sacred* science through a consciousness of the heart—an alignment with universal truth and knowledge. To quote Schwaller again:

> We have borrowed the term "intelligence-of-the-heart" from the ancient Egyptians in order to designate that other aspect of man which allows us to penetrate beyond our animal limits and which, in truth, makes for human man's characteristic progression toward divine Man: the awakening of this original principle that lies dormant in every living human being. Intelligence-of-the-heart is purely a function of experienced innate consciousness. (1960/1985, p. 13)

All that being said, it seems clear that the most probable place in our modern culture that we would find a consciousness of the heart is in spirituality. Even the traditional religions have at their mystic foundation a powerful commitment to what is morally sound and "right." This was and has been expressed in art, literature, and the architecture and construction of magnificent temples and cathedrals throughout the world since the inception of Judaism, Christianity, Islam, Hinduism, and Buddhism. With notable exceptions, one could argue that a major missing element in many of these dominant religious paradigms was an awareness of consciousness and soul in *all* things. Connection with the divine typically could only be found through the Church (in the Western traditions at least) and a sense of unity or even a relationship with God could not be individually found anywhere in nature or even within one's self. On a much smaller scale there have been numerous religious sects, secret societies, and seemingly cultish groups that have championed a form of consciousness of the heart as an important component of their core belief system. Many of these groups were successful at embodying basic tenets of the ancient Egyptian cosmology. None of them, however, ever came close to the massive following needed in order to create an entire community and culture around their doctrines. Many were persecuted by the major dominating religion of their place and time, and many were simply too obscure and out of touch with the basic mindset of the masses.

It seems, however, that the modern world is not completely devoid of a sacred science cosmology—but whatever there is of it appears weak, unorganized, unconscious, and without material intention. It is not difficult to find a *spiritual intention* in most modern as well as not-so-modern religious and spiritual disciplines. Material intention, however, seems to be essential for a sacred science to be fully realized. Yet, in our culture, the more material an intention is, the less likely a spiritual or deeply felt intelligence of the heart will be tolerated or even considered in executing that intention. Material intention is an intention to directly affect the material world through the mind or, more appropriately, considering the context of this book, through the soul, heart, or psyche—it is, as Schwaller said, a "relationship between the life in us and observation of that life in Nature" (1960/1985, p. 14). The word "nature" here would imply a physical reality. One popular explanation of this process is for mind to "think" of a mental equivalent of what is desired to manifest in the exterior world, and then soul, or consciousness of the heart, implements the manifestation. This material manifestation could consist of purely physical things, such as a body healing or material wealth, but a deeper and more meaningful endeavor would be toward more conscious relationships between individuals and communities, the expression of love in the world, global peace and prosperity, and a healthy planet. This would be a relationship between the life within us,[1] the life of *ma'at*, and the exterior life around us—the material world of form.

In recent years (since the late 19th century), a handful of spiritual movements seem to have had the ancient Egyptian sacred science at the heart of their doctrines. Before the theosophists, which is the first group I will discuss, there certainly were many spiritual groups, dogmas, and so forth that held a form of consciousness of the heart at the core of their belief systems. As mentioned earlier, probably all religious systems can be described as primarily heart conscious as opposed to head conscious—but this heart-conscious concept is interpreted quite differently in other religious doctrines. However, not until the turn of the century in the Western world did a concentrated focus on a material intention begin to form within a spiritual context—at least on a larger scale than levitations, materializations, and the like, which had been practiced in India and elsewhere in the world for centuries. This material intention can be described, in ancient Egyptian terms, as an effort to "do *ma'at*"—to create a material world in harmony with the inner world. Schwaller's consciousness of the heart was again an awareness of an innate alignment with "rightness." This consciousness was applied to all things, not just to love and moral concepts but also to architecture, medicine, and engineering. The beginnings of this shift in the late 18th century blossomed into modern groups that have a very powerful material intention evident in such diverse areas as mind body medicine, positive thinking, abundance consciousness, and manifestation through thought.

What most of these modern systems lack, however, are a large community, organization, discipline, and a unifying doctrine. They also are possibly *too* materially intended, individualistic, and egoistic and lack at their core (at least in common practice) a spiritual context of unity love and community compassion. (The ancient Egyptians did not necessarily find these attributes defining in their own cosmology but did devote their attention and effort to satisfying their gods and following the consciousness of the heart.) Many of these systems are driven by an egoistic passion for material acquisition through a fear of lack rather than being driven by a need and desire for an ordered external world reflecting the inner perfect world of *ma'at*.

Several larger movements, however, have been close to establishing a system of a universal nature that could be close to utilizing a more congruent form of the ancient Egyptian sacred science. I will proceed to present three of these systems: Madame Blavatsky's Theosophist movement of the late 19th and early 20th century; Rudolf Steiner's Anthroposophical Society; and the New Thought movement, which includes Charles and Myrtle Fillmore's Unity Church, Ernest Holmes's Church of Religious Science, and Mary Baker Eddy's Church of Christ, Scientist. I have chosen these three only as limited examples of modern systems that have some form of Schwaller's consciousness of the heart at the foundation of their belief system. Again, there are many more organizations such as these, and in our current time, we find more and more individuals embracing a heart consciousness as their own personal credo.

Helena Petrovna Blavatsky (1831–1891) was born in what is now Dnepropetrovsk, Ukraine. She eventually became a significant figure in the world of esoteric studies and spirituality. As mentioned earlier, Blavatsky believed the roots of all esoteric knowledge lay either in Tibet or ancient Egypt. Even as a young child, Blavatsky seemed destined for the life of an individual with an understanding and connection with the world around her. At an early age, she talked of inanimate objects such as stones or bits of dead twigs as having consciousness and told elaborate stories about the life of fossils she observed in the riverbed by her home as well as what she found in the Saratov museum. She had a fascination with the dead, told scary stories to the other children with whom she mingled, and was very likely considered a somewhat odd child.

As an adult, Blavatsky had a rather colorful life traveling around the world several times to such exotic places as India, Egypt, Greece, England, America, and Tibet (although it is not certain she actually made it to Tibet). Guided by the Masters, primarily two mystical adepts, Morya and Koot Hoomi, Blavatsky eventually established the Theosophical Society with Henry Steel Olcott and William Quan Judge in New York City in 1875. The major tenets of the society were to

> form a nucleus of the universal brotherhood of humanity without distinction of race, creed, sex, caste, or color, to encourage the study of comparative religion, philosophy, and science, and to investigate the unexplained laws of nature and the powers latent in man. (Blavatsky & Codd, 1953, p. 24)

Before establishing the society with its lofty mission, Blavatsky learned the mystical ways of the adepts through study with various mystics she encountered in her travels. In 1874, she met the journalist and lawyer Colonel Henry Steel Olcott while investigating a paranormal incident in Chittenden, New York. They became nearly inseparable friends for many years following their meeting and shared the vision and mission of the Theosophical Society. Olcott went on to become, in his later years, quite a celebrity himself among the Buddhists of Ceylon (now Sri Lanka) and elsewhere, championing their cause and assisting in their struggle to pull themselves out of political and spiritual despair through his efforts to instill pride and personal ownership of their ancient belief systems and Buddhist doctrines.

One of the primary inspirations for the establishment of a society of like-minded thinkers was a lecture Olcott, Blavatsky, and Judge attended, which was delivered in New York City by George H. Felt, an inventor, engineer, and architect who had been a member of the Miracle Club, a failed attempt by Olcott and Blavatsky to form a secret society, as suggested by the Masters, that would become a spiritual society. The title of Felt's lecture was "The Lost Canon of Proportion of the Egyptians, Greeks, and Romans" and it was held in Blavatsky's rooms in 1875. According to Gary Lachman (2012), a prominent biographer of Blavatsky, Felt claimed that:

> The men who designed the pyramids were adepts. Their great structures, which have survived millennia, were not made of only bricks and mortar—or the ancient Egyptian equivalent—but were the product of an occult wisdom, carefully guarded by the high priests. This wisdom consisted of an exact mystical science, which could be housed in specific geometric designs. (p. 130)

All three future theosophists in attendance, Blavatsky, Judge, and Olcott, were so inspired by the speech that they seemed to decide simultaneously that they must form the new theosophist society. Excitedly they passed notes to one another proclaiming their eagerness to engage in this joint pursuit, and soon after, the Theosophical Society was officially established. It is interesting to note that Felt's lecture appeared to be a clear forerunner to the conclusions reached by Schwaller de Lubicz more than sixty years later with his formulation of the ancient Egyptian concept of intelligence of the heart resulting from his rigorous investigation of the geometry of the Temple of Man in Luxor.

Several years after the establishment of the Theosophical Society in New York in 1875, Blavatsky and Olcott headed for Adyar, India and created a new international headquarters for the society there. Their close associate, William Quan Judge, an active lawyer cum mystic, was left behind to run the New York division. Over the ensuing years, the original Theosophical Society has split into several factions and is still active worldwide. Although their first primary mission—to prepare the public for a global spiritual leader surfacing in the world in the later part of the 20th century—essentially failed, Theosophists are still dedicated to the investigation of "unexplained laws of nature and the powers latent in man."

Blavatsky was quite a controversial figure. Her entry into the esoteric spiritual–religious world of the late 19th century coincided with the spiritualist movement of the same era. Spiritualism is a belief system and practice that holds to the conviction that deceased people can communicate with the living as spirits through audible means, the apportation and materialization of objects, and the creation of a substance commonly known in the spiritualist's world as *ectoplasm*. The spiritualist craze in the Western world lasted nearly eighty years and took America by storm. Although Blavatsky believed in the continuation of the spirit after death and even believed in many of the materializations that the mediums and psychics conjured up, she did not believe that the manifestations were coming from the actual spirit of the deceased. She argued that the true spirit moves on and is far too busy to play at parlor games with the living. Many of the prominent spiritualists of the day had issue with her opposition to their life's work and made great effort to discredit Blavatsky and expose her as the charlatan they believed she was.

Through her training by the Masters, Blavatsky became very adept at the mental manipulation of the material world herself. She allegedly created objects out of thin air, having caused bunches of roses to fall from the ceiling of her home onto the heads of her doubting guests and other objects to appear or to be found in unlikely places (such as a teacup and saucer that matched an existing service found buried in the ground surrounded by a tangle of tree roots). She was known to cause writing to appear mysteriously on paper and seemed to make jewelry disappear and rematerialize, rapping to occur, bells to tinkle, and flames to dim, among similar episodes. She did, however, grow tired of these displays and limited their frequency. She discounted these revelations as immature expressions devoid of any real meaning, which caused many devotees anxious for material demonstrations to become frustrated and leave the society. This lack of meaning in such feats is the primary reason she had such a negative view of the spiritualists, and they of her, and she called this sort of psychic demonstration the pinnacle of materialism—the very thing she wished to assuage.

Blavatsky's training in esoteric wisdom was extensive, and her writings throughout her career were copious and mammoth. Her seminal multivolume works, *The Secret Doctrine* (1888/1977) and *Isis Unveiled* (1877/1965), amount to over 2,500 pages combined. Again guided by the Masters, Blavatsky seemed to possess supernatural powers in her ability to quote extensively from works that were not readily at her disposal. She was a highly disciplined writer and spent the majority of each day with a pen in hand when she was immersed in the completion of her books. She believed she had a mission, and the Masters made it clear to her that this indeed was the truth, as she toiled often while in extremely ill health to accomplish her divine undertaking. Gary Lachman (2012) commented:

> When *Isis Unveiled* appeared, Western consciousness had entered a kind of metaphysical black hole. Although Christianity was still a powerful presence—hence Blavatsky's criticisms—it was fighting a losing battle against a reductive, exclusively materialist science, the conclusion of which was that the universe, and the life within it, were ultimately meaningless, an assessment it still stands by today. (p. 158)

Here, Lachman touched on a central tenet of ancient Egyptian cosmology, as stated by Blavatsky: "It is not spirit which dwells in matter, but matter which clings temporarily to spirit" (1877/1965, p. 428). This statement, from *Isis Unveiled*, was still possibly too dualistic for ancient Egyptian sensibilities—although when trying to recover from a dualist paradigm seated in a materialist worldview, as we are in this modern context, this becomes the clear manner in which to express this concept—in terms of matter and spirit being perceived as separate. Blavatsky continued: "No man, however gross and material he may be, can avoid leading a double existence; one in the visible universe, the other in the invisible" (p. 180). Lachman (2012) commented on this statement as well:

> This last remark is the central insight of *all* Hermetic, esoteric, occult, and spiritual philosophy: that human beings are the inhabitants of *two* worlds, the mundane world we unavoidably encounter every day, and *another* world, which transcends this one and in which we are not constrained by the usual limits of time and space. (p. 167)

Yes, in our current state of materialist blindness we would perceive this material, everyday world as mundane. But the ancient Egyptians very likely did not see the material world as anything other than a magical world bubbling with animated life, seen and unseen, "not constrained by the usual limits of time and space." We must try to comprehend what it would mean to be in a nondualistic reality where we did not discern the difference between the inner and outer world. The ancient Egyptians may have been able to distinguish a differing *quality* between their inner reality and their outer reality but probably not in a manner in which we, today, comprehend the "two" realities and their integration. Blavatsky as well as other spiritual adepts may have understood this clearly. However, as their writing and teaching was meant to inform a world ensconced in the limitations of an exclusively materialist reality, the language used had to conform to these limitations of perception.

Blavatsky died in 1891, leaving a confusing personal legacy. She was quite misunderstood by the general public, and due to several scathing biographies and more than a few legal battles regarding her authenticity, it is difficult to fashion a clear image of her personal character, values, and beliefs if one digs only a few inches below the surface of her biographical history. What is clear, however, is the legacy of her achievements in the esoteric, spiritual, foundations of her writing and in the work of the institution she helped found and create, the Theosophical Society. Still considered a powerful source of esoteric knowledge and practice, Theosophical Society lodges can be found in numerous countries still dedicated to the three tenets of the original institution.

Many great thinkers, philosophers, and spiritual men and women have been members of Blavatsky's society (including Thomas Edison, who was busy at one time developing a device to record spirit voices). One who was greatly influenced by the society, but never formally joined, was Rudolf Steiner, born in 1861 in what is now the northern part of Croatia. At the time of his birth, this place was part of the Austrian Empire. Steiner eventually founded the Anthroposophical Society in the early 20th century, which had at its foundation a belief in reincarnation and karma and was dedicated to goals similar to those found in Blavatsky's Theosophy: to pull modern humanity out of the downward spin of materialism and to bring humans' inner awareness in alignment with the greater awareness of the universe.

Steiner was greatly influenced by the celebrated minds of his era and times past, most notably Immanuel Kant, the famed German philosopher, who had died over a half century before Steiner's birth, and Johann Wolfgang von Goethe, a scientist and poet who formed much of Steiner's view that scientific observation and study retain a qualitative element rather than be wholly quantitative. In accord with the thesis of this book, Goethe and Steiner believed that soul had a place in the hard sciences as well as in art and religion. Steiner described his spiritual philosophy as *spiritual science.*

Steiner's effort to create an awareness of the unseen, spiritual world equal to humanity's awareness of the material, physical world is evident in the many physical-world endeavors that, to this day, define his legacy, including the Waldorf schools of education, biodynamic farming, and the Camphill Villages for adults with developmental disabilities, as well as alternative perspectives in architecture and medical science. Especially unique about Steiner's work was his insistence on integrating the inner and outer world, as he believed there was no way to understand either without the full intellectual awareness of the two. Gary Lachman (2007), who was Steiner's biographer as well, noted, "For Steiner—the best instrument for examining nature, or the manmade world, is the human mind itself, when, through a discipline of the imagination, the inner and the outer worlds are unified" (p. 44).

Although Steiner's spiritual foundation was essentially Christian (even though his views did diverge from traditional Christian thought), his interests did expand to include the mysteries of Egypt, as evidenced in his book, *Egyptian Myths and Mysteries* (1911/1971). Possibly much of his own formulated spiritual system was derived from his study of ancient Egypt. Lachman (2007) explained, "Steiner's fundamental idea is that, when we open our eyes, what we take to be a simple, immediate perception of the external world, is already infused with the content of our inner, spiritual world, our consciousness" (p. 94). He added, "What Steiner and his fellow Idealists are saying is that you would not even have an outside world unless you first had something inside" (p. 95). According to what has been presented in this book, these ideas are similar to ancient Egyptian concepts. Reality for the ancient Egyptians was as much inner and symbolic as it was outer and physical. Although Lachman's statement implies a cause-and-effect functionality, it seems that there was no linear concept of time and space in the ancient Egyptian cosmology and that the outer and inner world existed simultaneously, with no clear demarcation between the two.

Even if Steiner's Anthroposophy is not an accepted mainstream modality of psychotherapy per se, the principles he presented regarding spiritual practice are noticeably similar to the concept presented in this book regarding an acceptance of the inner world equal to the materialist acceptance of the physical outer world. Steiner's material success in implementing this philosophy and spiritual practice is evident in the aforementioned areas of human endeavor, education, agriculture, and even medical science, just as the ancient Egyptians' success in the material world is evident in their extant monuments. Steiner's Anthroposophy, as compared to Blavatsky's Theosophy, had a more powerful and conscious material intention. Steiner was wholly dedicated to the application of his spiritual paradigm to the everyday affairs of human beings—in the education of children, the production of food, the creation of art and physical structures, and in medicine and health. Although it is doubtful that Steiner consciously developed his systems based on Egyptian sacred science concepts, he certainly utilized these concepts in formulating his spiritual schema.

Steiner also believed there were highly advanced civilizations before the Egyptians, at a time when the Earth, its surface, and even the physical construction of the beings that held "human" souls were radically different. The first civilization he described is Lemuria, an ancient lost continent that precedes Atlantis. Steiner did not invent Lemuria; it was originally proposed in 1864 by a zoologist, Philip Sclater, suggesting the origins of the lemur, a strepsirrhini primate found in Madagascar. Quite a few other occultists had theories about the people that populated Lemuria—Blavatsky, in particular, found a discussion of Lemuria and the Root Races found there (the Third Root Race) in the *Book of Dzyan*, a tome introduced to her by her Masters. As with Steiner, Blavatsky believed that God was disappointed with Lemuria and sank it into the sea, making way for Atlantis. Atlantis did not fare much better, and ultimately, it fell out of God's graces and also vanished into the ocean.

Needless to say, Steiner was not the first to mention Atlantis either, but he did have some rather differing opinions of what Atlantis and the Atlanteans were. He envisioned Atlantis as being an immense landmass, occupying most of what is now the Atlantic Ocean. He saw the people that occupied this land as highly integrated with nature and possessing and utilizing inner spiritual ways of perception and communication. He believed that Atlantean cities were built partially of intertwining trees that housed the inhabitants, all deeply fused with nature and the natural infrastructure. Although there has been no scientific discovery that corroborates Steiner's visions, many clairvoyants and spiritual women and men such as Edgar Cayce have had similar interpretations of Atlantis and her fate. Cayce (1877–1945), an American psychic whose predictive powers and insights into the distant past were astonishing to other spiritual minds of the time, described Atlantis's structure, inhabitants, spiritual systems, and other attributes almost exactly as Steiner had.

Steiner died in 1925, leaving behind a legacy that is still contributing to the whole of modern culture. As mentioned earlier, his Waldorf schools continue to practice Steiner's educational methodology, bringing more imagination into education. Biodynamic farming as a holistic understanding of agriculture and other Steiner-inspired insights into medicine, architecture, dance, music, and art are still utilized and honored through a variety of physical expressions. Steiner's core philosophy—a method to integrate a spiritual science into the mainstream of human culture—is probably the philosophy in current practice that is closest to a similar ancient Egyptian cosmology. In the following chapter, I examine in more detail the relationship between Steiner's spiritual worldview and Carl Jung's psychological model, as I bring psychology and a personal psychotherapy into the narrative.

The beginnings of the New Thought spiritual movement in the United States during the mid-19th century are usually attributed to Phineas Parkhurst Quimby (1802–1866). Quimby was a healer and one of the first in this country to proclaim that the mind and the body are connected and that it is possible for the mind to effectuate physical change in the body. Quimby believed that he had learned the secrets of Jesus and could heal people according to their beliefs. In 1859, he wrote an article entitled "Is Disease a Belief?" and in it proclaimed that "all sickness is in the mind or belief. . . . To cure the disease is to correct the error, and as disease is what follows the error, destroy the cause, and the effect will cease" (1921, p. 186).

With regard to the etiology of disease, Quimby clearly stated throughout his career that thought precedes form; cause comes before effect, and cause always has its roots in the mind. Quimby was a scientist at heart and had been trained as a skilled clockmaker. He proclaimed that his healing modality was solidly scientific but, when asked where the foundation of this science lay, also responded that Jesus the Christ was the first to understand and use this power. He used the phrase *Christian Science* before Mary Baker Eddy, the founder of the religious movement of Christian Science, popularized the term. Although much of Quimby's work was centered in a scientific model, he did consider his practice to be spiritually based and religious in nature.

Quimby's (1921) belief that the individual's power over the body lies in the individual's own belief system was integral to the healing process he utilized. He not only stated that belief is the cause of disease but also posited that most beliefs people possess are false, a view that assumes that there is a right way to be; in his context, *right* is to be disease free. If being disease free is to be in correct or true form, then the subject's belief in disease must be a false belief, an error in thinking, or "false reasoning" (p. 295). Quimby stated, "Disease is something made by belief or forced upon us by our parents or public opinion. . . . Now if you can face the error and argue it down then you can cure the sick" (pp. 173–174). Quimby's insistence that a belief could be either *false* or *correct* was based on his assumption that God intends for humans to live a life of perfect health and happiness and that their belief, in order to be *correct*, should be congruent with God's intentions (which certainly sounds congruent with the consciousness of the heart). His scientific reasoning would more than likely not have supported such a judgment regarding the purpose of human existence and God's desire to see his human subjects live in a world of perfect bliss. Although one could argue that disease has as much of a right to exist and evolve in the world as humankind, Quimby's position resonates with the divine concept that benevolence is *a priori* in the universe and that the closer mankind gets to a full awareness of oneness and unity, the less need there will be for disease and suffering (Braden, 1987).

Certainly, it takes little effort to correlate the Egyptian concept of *ma'at*, the ultimate divine balance and norm, with Quimby's concept of *false belief* and God's will that human beings, in their "true" expression, are disease free. Although the Egyptians may not have been as concerned about the physical body being "perfect" during the time of the spirit's physical occupation, they did seem to see the body as occupying several states of expression simultaneously, and one of those states could be as disease free, or more accurately, devoid of physical defect. The meticulous way they prepared their kings and royalty for the afterlife, with food, chariots, personal items, and, in the Old Kingdom, even servants and attendants present in their burial crypts, is a testament to this "mixed" way of perceiving reality. Was it merely a superstitious belief that their dead kings would rise again and rule the physical land, or was it an understanding that as they honored the physical with attention and conscious intention they would also honor the spiritual world where their kings actually did express their existence, in some "form," again or even simultaneously?

Quimby was reportedly the teacher and mentor of several other prominent New Thought leaders. Mary Baker Eddy visited him as a patient several years before his death in 1866. At that time, she was nearly an invalid, and almost immediately after following Quimby's methods of healing, she became rid of her ailments. Warren Felt Evans, considered the first chronicler of New Thought, and Julius and Annetta Dresser, ardent followers of Quimby in their own spiritual healing practice, were but a few other patients of Quimby who went on to further the cause of New Thought. Mary Baker Eddy eventually founded the Church of Christ, Scientist and also was the one-time mentor of Emma Curtis Hopkins, who is considered the modern founder of the New Thought movement and is attributed with teaching or influencing several of New Thought's most prominent practitioners. Among them are Myrtle and Charles Fillmore, the founders of the modern Christian Church, Unity, and Ernest Holmes, the founder of Science of Mind and the Church of Religious Science (now carrying the more upbeat moniker, Centers for Spiritual Living). Eddy eventually split from the general group of New Thought ideology and became in conflict with many of its practitioners, including Hopkins.

Although the New Thought movement was originally obsessed with physical healing, much of its underlying philosophy came out of the work of Ralph Waldo Emerson (1944). Emerson was a contemporary of Quimby, born in 1803 and died in 1882, and was responsible for pushing Western culture a tad further away from the oppression of religious dogma with his emphasis on transcendentalism and individuality. He was one of the first prominent writers to expound upon the divinity of man and individual, personal, Christ Consciousness. Most of the New Thought pioneers, in particular, Ernest Holmes, saw Emerson and his humanistic philosophy a cornerstone to the movement.

Holmes based much of his philosophy on Emerson's work. He also studied the works of Thomas Troward (1904, 1991), a scientist who wrote extensively on the concept of the *Law*. This Law refers to the workings of mind-to-body manifestation—or the psyche-to-matter issue. According to Troward and others in the New Thought arena, the Law is impersonal and functions according to very strict rules of thought and intention. It has no care as to whether the operator who puts the law into motion suffers as a result or not. The Law is simply the law, and creates whatever is asked of it. Troward warned against being unaware of thought processes such as those that are constantly whirring around in a person's unconscious mind. He claimed that the Law responds to *any* thought, whether conscious or not, and for people to maintain any sort of control over their experience, they must train their minds to think only of what they wish to materialize in their lives. Ernest Holmes (1938) borrowed from Troward's writings, but also presented the idea that trained thought is far more powerful than untrained thought, meaning that casual and simplistic thinking will not have as much affect as disciplined and intentional thinking.

The common thread running through the work of all of these practitioners and mental healers is their adherence to Quimby's original idea that the body is directly influenced by the mind—or, considering the context of this book, that the physical world is *directly* influenced, and even created, by the mind. This axiom of Quimby's need not be applied only to physical healing but also to the entire world of effect. Beneath this mechanical function of mind–body interaction, there is the power of spiritual or divine guidance and intention. Quimby believed that a physical result that is undesired is produced from a belief, which, in its very inception, is false (possibly not in alignment with *ma'at*?). He and the men and women of New Thought that followed him believed that the very essence of self is divine spirit and thus is immutable. This spirit can only *know* the Truth, and the Truth can never be threatened by anything. The *realness* of this *a priori* essence of spirit is the only thing that can truly exist; therefore, anything contrary to it is false, or *unreal*. In this regard, disease does not even exist.

Ernest Holmes created what he considered a scientific method for bringing about physical change in a person's life—or a formula for manifestation. The basic tenet of this method was "let it be done to you according to your belief" (Matthew 8:13, King James Version). Holmes said that the universe would never deny humans anything unless they believed that the universe was incapable of supplying it. He felt that the seed of belief has to be planted in the mind in order for the mind to maintain the spiritual truth that the universe is unlimited and is the abundant source of all of human desire. Holmes claimed that the material mechanism that can bring a desire into form is of no real concern and, in fact, is God's job to implement. Holmes believed the intellect is limited by a materialist perception of reality and that belief has to come from the heart, not the intellect. The planting of this seed of belief, he proposed, is accomplished through the *spiritual mind treatment.* This is a type of prayer that affirms the truth as a present reality rather than as something to be desired and attained in the future. According to Holmes, the spiritual mind treatment thus sets into motion the resonating alignment with the all-potential nature of the universe. It makes specific what is desired from this soup of infinite mind and then brings this desire into form by insisting on its already apparent reality.

As early as 1938, Holmes was implying that time is not a reality and insisting that effective prayer rely on the acceptance that all that is desired already exists, regardless of the illusion of appearance. Although the spiritual mind treatment was created to effect change in one's life, it is clear that Holmes contended that one's life is already whole and complete in the mind of God—the *timeless* mind of God. Holmes taught that cause and effect is the operation of the Law, but with his idea of affirming in prayer the acceptance of the desired effect as being wholly present in the *now*, Holmes was in fact denying the existence of past and future.

Holmes (1938) believed in holding in thought the truth that is God and thus forming a *mental equivalent* of that truth. This is more than merely visualization, although visualizing a desire is certainly a proposed method of bringing thought into form. Holmes believed, however, that it is more than the visual idea or imagined object in the mind's eye that brings about the effect in the world. He believed that alignment with the spiritual truth or spiritual principle behind the desire is the real catalyst that puts the Law in motion. In fact, he insisted that this spiritual principle is always present, completely and in its entirety, at any given moment. A person's belief in or awareness of the spiritual principle thus brings about the form to represent it. If it is success that a person desires, it is in fact the *feeling* of success that they are truly holding to. The spiritual principle behind success, said Holmes, is abundance, happiness, and joy. Holmes suggested that, through spiritual treatment, a person holds in their thought the mental equivalent of these principles and that the universe will form before their eyes the appearance of what they physically equate with success. He stated:

> Since we are dealing with an Infinite Power, which knows only Its own ability to do, and since It can objectify any idea impressed upon It, there can be no limit to what It can or would do for us, other than the limit of our inward embodiment. *Limitation is not in Principle nor in Law, but only in the individual use we make of Principle.* Our individual use of It can only equal our individual capacity to understand It, to embody It. We cannot demonstrate beyond our ability to provide a mental equivalent of our desire. (p. 119)

Obviously none of these ideas was new with Ernest Holmes or any of the other practicing New Thought spiritual seekers. Jesus (who many scholars believe was trained by priests in ancient Egypt) is probably the most widely known practitioner of this science of mind, but clearly, other religious precedents to this belief system have existed. The Buddhists, for example, follow a tenet declaring that all that we are is the result of what we have thought: it is founded on our thoughts and is made up of our thoughts. If a person speaks or acts with an evil thought, pain follows that person, as the wheel follows the foot of the ox that draws the carriage (Lin, 1943, p. 13). This concept is not wholly original with Buddhism either. Much of this philosophy can be found in ancient Hinduism as well. We can also see it, if we tilt our heads a bit, in the ancient Egyptian concept of *ma'at*. As noted earlier, *ma'at* denotes the concept of divine perfection, order, and truth. Holmes and the other New Thought devotees believed that "Absolute Truth" was the Truth of God—perfect, creative, and life giving. Regardless of what a person experienced in the physical realm, the Absolute Truth behind it was the only Truth there was. All the rest, if it did not match Absolute Truth, was illusion, or simply relative truths (lower-case truth). Disease, because it does not match perfection, pure creativity, and life, was considered an "appearance"—a relative truth, but ultimately an illusion. If a person who is diseased were to see beyond the appearance, the disease would disappear.

Much New Thought literature stresses the point that all thought is power and that all thought is acted upon by the Law. Thomas Troward, in *The Edinburgh and Doré Lectures on Mental Science*, stated:

> We must therefore always be very clear as to whether we are *consciously* using first cause or not. Note the word "consciously" because, whether consciously or unconsciously, we are always using first cause; and it was for this reason I emphasized the fact that the Universal Mind is purely subjective and therefore bound by the laws which apply to subjective mind on whatever scale. Hence we are *always* impressing some sort of ideas upon it, whether we are aware of the fact or not, and all our existing limitations result from our having habitually impressed upon it that idea of limitation which we have imbibed by restricting all possibility to the region of secondary causes. (1904, pp. 57–58)

As stated previously, however, according to Ernest Holmes, trained thought is always more powerful than untrained thought, but it is equally important to note that trained thought can also reside in the unconscious and thus not be consciously known. Trained thought, or trained belief, can also reside in the collective unconscious or even in the cell memory of the body. It is ultimately one's own higher conscious awareness that brings any of these thoughts to the surface as a choice, or an accepted reality. All thought can manifest, and according to Quimby and others of the New Thought movement, all thought *will* manifest. It is the responsibility of the conscious mind, however, to accept the appearance presented in front of it as being congruent or incongruent with its own belief. It is easy to accept any physical appearance as real and as believable; after all, it is one's own beliefs that put it there in the first place. Material reality is also a cunning seducer, but what is the harm in accepting a manifestation that seems agreeable and pleasant? None whatsoever, as long as a person is not attached to its apparent reality. If a person is attached, the attachment simply limits his or her experience. The point is, as Jesus stressed so many years ago, people have *choice*, regardless of the appearance: "Judge not according to the appearance, but judge righteous judgment" (John 7:24).

New Thought is a belief system that relies on the Absolute Truths of God—essentially that love and creativity are at the center of reality—the power of thought that precedes form, and the Law (the combination of thought and Truth) to execute the manifestation of material reality. The fundamental obligation of those following this belief system is to align themselves with Truth (which we could relate to *ma'at*) and thus effectuate a mirroring of the Truths of God from an internal locus to an external, material reality. This is a crude explanation but acceptably clear on most crucial points.

All three of these systems, Theosophy, Anthroposophy, and New Thought, share several vital tenets, the foremost being a desire within the system to expand human awareness to an unseen and "in the mind" (or heart, or even "mind of God") source that is as important, if not more important, than the limited physical outer world. Each had its own individual method to execute this basic foundational tenet. Blavatsky hoped for a transcendent connection with her fellow humans through a disciplined study and practice of the occult mysteries; Steiner wanted to apply this fuller awareness of the nonmaterial side of reality to an effective and useful manipulation of the physical world in farming, education, and medicine; and New Thought focused, at least initially, on healing the physical body but expanded into a promotion of love and unity through physical creativity, abundance (in all things desired that are in alignment with Absolute Truth—again, a consciousness of the heart), and happiness. Although none of them specifically used any Egyptian ritual or doctrine, each did recognize the ancient traditions of Egypt as well as other traditions as a prominent origin of their underlying dogmas.

As mentioned previously, there have been dozens if not hundreds of philosophies, belief systems, religions, and other groups that have utilized a sort of consciousness of the heart in the expression and execution of their doctrines. The three briefly outlined here are simply examples of recent major efforts to break out of the shadowy limits of materialist thought. Since the Age of Enlightenment in the 18th century, science has been the sole arbiter of truth in Western culture, with its reductionist and quantifying method of demonstrating credibility for varied theories regarding nature and how the universe functions. Theosophy, Anthroposophy, and New Thought were three major efforts that challenged the reining scientific definition of reality and sought to bring back to humanity an esoteric, occult, and ancient perspective of the universe and our place within it. They endeavored to reawaken the sleeping soul in our modern materialist paradigm and bring a consciousness of the heart to the forefront of human awareness.

Note

1 The life within us being of an "inner nous or sacred knowingness that will result in a greater balance and alignment with harmony and evolutionary growth" (Chapter 1)

References

Blavatsky, H. (1965). *Isis unveiled*. Pasadena, CA: Theosophical University Press. (Original work published 1877)

Blavatsky, H. (1977). *The secret doctrine*. Pasadena, CA: Theosophical University Press. (Original work published 1888)

Blavatsky, H., & Codd, C. M. (1953). *The key to theosophy*. Adyar, Madras: Theosophical Pub. House.

Braden, C. (1987). *Spirits in rebellion: The rise and development of new thought*. Dallas, TX: Southern Methodist University Press.

Emerson, R. W. (1944). *The essays of Ralph Waldo Emerson*. New York, NY: Barnes.

Holmes, E. (with Lathem, M. A.). (1938). *The science of mind* (Completely revised and enlarged ed.). New York, NY: McBride.

Lachman, G. (2007). *Rudolf Steiner: An introduction to his life and work*. New York, NY: Tarcher/Penguin.

Lachman, G. (2012). *Madame Blavatsky: The mother of modern spirituality*. New York, NY: Tarcher/Penguin.

Lin, Y. (1943). *Between tears and laughter*. New York, NY: Day.

Quimby, P. (1921). *The Quimby manuscripts* (H. Dresser, Ed.). New York, NY: Crowell.

Schwaller de Lubicz, R. A. (1985). *Esoterism and symbol* (A. VandenBroeck & G. VandenBroeck, Trans.). New York, NY: Inner Traditions International. (Original work published 1960)

Steiner, R. (1971). *Egyptian myths and mysteries: Twelve lectures, Leipzig, September 2–14, 1908* (N. MacBeth, Trans.). New York, NY: Anthroposophic Press. (Original work published 1911)

Troward, T. (1904). *The Edinburgh and Doré lectures on mental science*. Marina Del Rey, CA: DeVorss.

Troward, T. (1991). *The creative process in the individual*. Marina del Rey, CA: DeVorss.

7

JUNGIAN PSYCHOLOGY AND THE SEARCH FOR SOUL

Many people surrounding Carl Gustav Jung, and many who came after him, considered him a mystic, and there is probably no other label he detested more. Jung thought of himself as an empirical scientist and believed all of his conclusions and theories to be thoroughly seated in scientific methodology—at least that is what he said. It mattered greatly to Jung that people, at least the important and influential people in his life, believed he was a scientist and a serious medical psychiatrist. Jung made great effort to obscure his passion for things supernatural and mystical, but he didn't do such a great job of it. Being a respected scientist was important to him, and essential to his prominent, and serious, standing in the community. However, it was clear from his writing and his work, and certainly made more clear when his manuscript, *The Red Book* (2009), was finally released to the public decades after his death, that Jung had some rather mystical ideas.

These ideas were always on the edge, at best, and he often had a difficult time keeping his enthusiasm for things considered unscientific from leaking through his writing and lectures. He parted with his primary professional and personal mentor, Sigmund Freud, due to disagreements regarding their respective theories of the unconscious. Freud always preferred to stick to a purely scientific explanation for his own ideas and argued that Jung's theories were a bit on the mystic and spiritual side of things. Jung did argue, for example, that his theory of the collective unconscious—innate propensities and patterns that all humans from every culture throughout history shared—was a scientific fact, whereas Freud found it a tad supernatural and more of a spiritual and metaphysical concept than a scientific one.

Recall Marie-Louise von Franz's comments cited in Chapter 4 regarding Jung's insistence that a patient of his had actually been on the moon in her psychical world, and that the physical moon familiar to us in our material reality is actually the illusion (Whitney & Whitney, 1986). Recall as well, in the same chapter, Jung's conversation with his pots and pans at Bollingen. Jung did seem to believe in a connection between the psyche and the physical world and did, as a result, step into the realm of the supernatural. After all, there is no known operating conduit between matter and the mind, and certainly none that material science can attest to.

Jung's earlier days are also filled with experiences and pursuits that would classify him as a mystic, with ideas and beliefs that are in alignment with sacred science and the consciousness of the heart. In *Jung the Mystic* (Lachman, 2010), much is revealed about Jung's efforts to remain the objective medical doctor and scientist in the public eye and suppress whatever mystical beliefs and understandings he may have held: "Jung seemed to have two minds about the supernatural: a public one that wanted to understand it 'scientifically,' and a private one that acknowledged ghosts, visions, and premonitions as part of the essential mystery of life" (p. 4). It is again apparent from Jung's interests and the topics he chose to write about that he had a prevailing fascination with the occult and parapsychology. Jung attended séances from an early adult age and had interest in the paranormal due to (among other influences) a grandfather who talked to his dead wife and a mother who had several noticeable personality quirks and could have, at times, been channeling entities from the spirit world. Jung's (1961/1963) own autobiographical endeavor, *Memories, Dreams, Reflections*, exposed much of his spiritual side, but he was careful to keep this spirituality tucked safely away in his psychology. As mentioned before, it was not until the publication of his extensive, illustrated journal, *The Red Book* (2009), that a clear materialization of the inner world of Jung appeared through his art and writing.

Due to this sort of split personality—scientist and mystic—Jung often wrote in circles and many times the presentation of his ideas was confusing and contradictory. One of Jung's (1931/1964) most interesting essays that relates to the subject of primitive culture, written at a time when ancient Egypt would have been considered such a culture, is "Archaic Man," in which he discussed many of the conclusions he drew after visiting East Africa and conversing with the primal tribes of that area in 1925. He presented several ideas in this essay, among them the suggestion that the primitive human is nonpsychological and assumes reality to be a representation of his or her own psychic world. Jung describes this as a projection. In the early pages of his essay, Jung considered this essentially to be a problem, as he claimed:

> It is a rational presupposition of ours that everything has a natural and perceptible cause. We are convinced of this right from the start. Causality is one of our most sacred dogmas. There is no legitimate place in our world for invisible, arbitrary and so-called supernatural forces. (p. 54 [*Collected Works* ('*CW*') 10, para. 113])

In a clause attached to the last sentence, he continued his thought with a comment about quantum science, introducing a bit of a doubt concerning the rationality of his causality statement: "unless, indeed, we descend with the modern physicist into the obscure, microcosmic world inside the atom, where, it appears, some very curious things happen" (p. 54 [*CW* 10, para. 113]). Jung did not, at least in this essay, shed any further light on these "curious things."

Jung (1931/1964) continued with this idea of psychic projection as reality and, as such, a pathology:

> If an important psychic component is projected on a human being, he becomes *mana*, extraordinarily effective—a sorcerer, witch, werewolf, or the like. The primitive idea that the medicine-man catches the souls that have wandered away by night and puts them in cages like birds is a striking illustration of this. These projections give the medicine-man his mana, they cause animals, trees and stones to speak, and because they are his own psychic components they compel the projicient to obey them absolutely. For this reason an insane person is hopelessly at the mercy of his voices; they are projections of his own psychic activity whose unconscious subject he is. He is the one who speaks through his voices, just as he is the one who hears, sees and obeys. (p. 68 [*CW* 10, para. 137])

Jung was struggling with pathologizing the primitive medicine man's psychic projection, comparing it to the insane person being "hopelessly at the mercy of his voices." This seems eerily reminiscent of Jung's alleged speech to the pots and pans in his Bollingen kitchen and von Franz's interview comment, in the film *Matter of Heart* (Whitney & Whitney, 1986), that the psyche communicates with matter—not as a projection, but matter as a reality with its own autonomous being.

In the final pages of his essay, Jung (1931/1964) posed this question:

> Shall we, for the moment at least, venture the hypothesis that the primitive belief in arbitrary powers is justified by the facts and not merely from a psychological point of view? This sounds alarming, but I have no intention of jumping from the frying-pan into the fire and trying to prove that witchcraft actually works. (pp. 68–69 [*CW* 10, para. 139])

Notably, Jung is again careful to present delicately this idea of witchcraft actually working. Considering what is known of Jung presently, he possibly did believe this, at least from the perspective of external reality having a certain independence, objectivity, and autonomy. He continued with this conclusion in the form of these profound questions:

> The question is nothing less than this: Does the psychic in general—the soul or spirit or the unconscious—originate in us, or is the psyche, in the early stages of conscious evolution, actually outside us in the form of arbitrary powers with intentions of their own, and does it gradually take its place within us in the course of psychic development? (p. 69 [*CW* 10, para. 140])

These questions obviously raise other questions, and from the perspective of this book, show a relation between Jung's thought and the ancient Egyptian cosmology. The ancient Egyptians did seem to believe that the power and qualitative value of the material external world was possessed by that world and not created by human consciousness; for example, the sun itself was beautiful, the human psyche did not make it so—but what of the idea that humans' consciousness creates the reality around them? The foregoing statement reflects a dualistic perspective that separates human consciousness from material reality. The truth about unity consciousness, and how, within this unity concept, physical matter and psyche relate to one another, either as projection or independent reality, may be, as Schwaller de Lubicz (1963/1985) said, "absolute reality, not to be grasped by our intelligence" (p. 11). As discussed earlier, the psyche-to-matter issue—form coming forth from mind—relies on a linear time construct. It is difficult to say if the ancient Egyptians perceived the outer world as a *result* of the inner world, although that is the only way we now would be able to comprehend it.

Along this train of thought, it is impossible to ignore the work of Jung in collaboration with the eminent physicist of his time, Wolfgang Pauli (Pauli & Jung, 2001). Although possibly more appropriate as part of the discussion in Chapter 4, "The Psyche-to-Matter Problem," here is where a distinct overlap exists, as the material pertaining to Pauli and Jung can easily be viewed as psychological but also clearly relates to quantum physics, science, and materialism.

As documented by Jungian analyst David Lindorff (2004, p. 26), in his book, *Pauli and Jung: The Meeting of Two Great Minds*, Pauli became aware of Jung's psychological theories when he sought therapy due to a severe emotional breakdown following his divorce in 1930. Both Pauli and Jung lived near Zurich at the time, and Pauli's father suggested that he visit Jung for analysis. Pauli became familiar with some of the basics of Jung's theories through attending some local lectures. Upon their first meeting, Jung suggested that Pauli consult with one of his pupils, a woman named Erna Rosenbaum, due to the fact that Pauli's issue seemed essentially to be his difficulty with women.

The focus of history and philosophy of science scholar Arthur Miller's (2010) *137: Jung, Pauli, and the Pursuit of Scientific Obsession* is Jung and Pauli's mutual effort to discover the cosmic number or *fine structure constant*, which is a fundamental physical constant dealing with electromagnetism or, from a different perspective, what could be considered the philosopher's stone of the mathematical universe. This was indeed one of Pauli and Jung's collaborative passions, but it was not the only concentration of their relationship. Quantum physics could be seen as the natural progression from ancient alchemy, through chemistry, culminating in the abstract world of subatomic particles, wave functions, and mathematics. Pauli was an eccentric scientist in this regard—he saw his scientific study to be directly related to Jung's study of the psyche. Miller's analysis of the content of their collaboration presents an informative introduction to the relationship between these men as well as deep exploration of their individual personal lives and perspectives. According to Miller, when Pauli underwent Jungian analysis for personal dysfunctions that had become insurmountable, he became fascinated with Jung's theories. He was mystified by how precisely the analysis and the theories behind it matched his own personal experience, which led him to study Jung's ideas about archetypes, typology, and alchemy. They soon began to exchange principle ideas from their own areas of expertise.

The correspondence between Pauli and Jung (2001) can be found in *Atom and Archetype*. Edited by Jungian psychologist C. A. Meier, this volume contains the letters of Jung and Pauli between 1932 and 1958. Also included are several essays about Jung and Pauli as well as several of their own and other pertinent letters and articles written by various authors. These works shed light on the integration of Jung's and Pauli's brilliance and knowledge in their respective fields—one being abstract internal imagery and the other being mathematical objectivity. Thomas Elsner, a Jungian analyst on the faculty at Pacifica Graduate Institute, suggested that Jung and Pauli were "tunneling through to the center of the same mountain from two different sides" (personal correspondence, June 3, 2013).

In his book, Lindorff (2004) went into further detail regarding the immersion of these two personalities into the problems of psyche and matter. He investigated the motivation of Pauli to connect with Jung's psychology and said:

> Physics was for him a way of probing into the very heart of nature. Like the alchemist, who saw images that reflected his inner self within the mysterious chemical transformations, Pauli thought of modern physics as a way station on the path to higher consciousness, "a way to salvation." (p. 80)

He observed that "Pauli believed there was an inner as well as an outer way of connecting to reality, and that these two options needed to be harmonized" (p. 81). With this reasoning, a connection to ancient Egyptian cosmology can be made whereby physics, spirituality, and psychology can possibly find a common patch of ground to stand on. Pauli's idea seems to be precisely what the ancient Egyptians were capable of doing and could possibly be seen as a definition of their sacred science: a harmonized inner and outer reality.

Lindorff observed that Pauli was quite interested in his own dreams and what their analysis could reveal to him, especially regarding physical symbolism. The analysis of his dreams and how they related to his study in quantum physics was a large part of his relationship with Jung. Over time, Pauli devised his own system of dream analysis, which was apparently not in agreement with Jung's; however, "their common interest in the deeper problem of the relationship between psyche and matter held them together" (2004, p. 81).

The article "Imagination as Laboratory," authored by Jungian analyst Beverley Zabriskie (2004), relates to this current book through its discussion of the imagination as the foundation for all material manifestation as well as for simple human *being* and relationship. She wrote:

> From psyche's perspective, the manifold forms of human registration and expression are both inward avenues into the complexities of being human, and outward vectors of entry into the structures of external reality. The symbolic and scientific both employ imagination. The human links emotion to imagination, and emotion makes imagination a matter of heart as well as mind. Imagination is thus a laboratory in science and psychology, for invention and discovery, for existence and emergence, for personhood and relationship. It may also prove to be a crucial conduit in relations among peoples, and thus for survival. (p. 4)

From a more contemporary perspective, this article supports Schwaller de Lubicz's (1963/1982) notion of the intelligence of the heart and presents imagination, the inner unseen world, as at least an equal partner in the creation of the external material world.

Although it might be appropriate to consider Jung a mystic, would it be appropriate to think of a form of Jungian psychology as a spiritual psychology? Jung did see a deeper meaning in being a human being than simply the machinations of a complex set of psychological functions. If a person's definition of "spiritual" is broad, then certainly any form of transcendent or even person-centered psychology could be considered spiritual. If we define "spiritual" to include an importance in the unseen world, then we could also consider Jung's efforts to shed meaningful light on the unconscious aspects of his patients as being a spiritual pursuit. To be spiritual, does a psychology need to focus on a supreme being such as God, or a variety of gods? Buddhists are known for not believing in what other religions define as "God," yet Buddhism is considered by most to be a spiritual system. It is beyond the scope of this book to engage in the debate about the existence of God or some unifying higher power that has intention and agenda in the creation and functioning of the universe (although it is true that consciousness of the heart implies a preconceived set order to the universe). What is important here is an acknowledgment and conscious use of a reality that is beyond the material reality modern science has told us is the only reality we need to contend with. If we can broaden our definition of spirituality to include this very basic, simple definition, then we can be assured that the ancient Egyptian cosmology and concept of consciousness of the heart is indeed spiritual. Jungian psychology in particular, and depth psychology in general, could then be classified as a spiritual psychology.

To delve deeper into this classification of spiritual psychology, a consideration of its roots in ancient traditions and religious beliefs is necessary. This idea is most evident in some of the earliest extant texts such as the *Corpus Hermeticum* (Copenhaver, 1992), a set of 20 books attributed to Hermes Trismegistus, known as the Thrice Great Hermes, as well as the pyramid texts and other Indian, Chinese, Mesopotamian, Hebrew, and Greek texts. The *Corpus Trismegistus* texts may predate the earliest-known editions, which were brought to Florence, Italy, by the monk Leonardo of Pistoia in 1460. These manuscripts were in Greek, and Cosimo de' Medici, the ruler of Florence, had such a thirst for knowledge that he instructed his trusted scholar Marsilio Ficino to stop work on his translation of Plato's dialogues and begin immediately on the translation of these mysterious works. These 20 volumes suffered much debate and controversy as they were thought to be originally attributed to the ancient Pharaohs' wisdom tradition. In them, Hermes, the Greek version of the Egyptian God Thoth, discusses with his disciple the source of all that is of, and in, the universe. *The Way of Hermes* (Salaman, van Oyen, Wharton, & Mahe, 2001) is a fine translation of these dialogues and contributes much to the understanding of this ancient wisdom.

Several other texts discussing Hermes and his influence on the Egyptian spiritual paradigm are relevant to this book. *The Hermetica* (Freke & Gandy, 2008) is a thorough and illuminating translation and interpretation of the *Corpus Hermeticum*. Although it is still debatable whether the *Corpus Hermeticum* is of ancient Egyptian origin, the earliest Egyptian texts, the pyramid texts, contain many passages almost identical to what is found in this ancient writing (Lachman, 2011). Fundamental to the message of the *Corpus Hermeticum* is that God is One and represents a unity consciousness in its creation of the universe and all that it contains. God is held to be the creator of both the material world and the inner world of thought. "God is both the material objects around us and the immaterial thoughts in our minds" (Freke & Gandy, 2008, p. 18). This ancient concept again dissolves the duality present in modern thinking, whereby the material world is assumed as somehow separate from the inner world of thought and as the only expression of reality.

The link between science and spirituality is evident in the Hermes texts. As the ancient Egyptians saw it, the two were not divided. "For Hermes, spiritual philosophy is not opposed to science, as it often is for us today. The student of spiritual philosophy studies science as a form of devotion to God" (Freke & Gandy, 2008, p. 1). In material, mechanistic, modern culture:

> people have ceased to see the universe as a source of wonder, and no longer revere it as the work of God. Spirituality has come to be dismissed by science as primitive superstition. The profound wisdom of the ancient Egyptians is thought of as a dead religion and as little more than an archaeological curiosity. Hermes foretells that Egypt, once the home of spirituality, will become a desolate place deserted by the gods. (Freke & Gandy, 2008, p. 2)

Hermes's prediction was that the world would become desolate and deserted by God (or "the gods") if spirituality were dismissed, as it fundamentally has been today. This essentially then becomes the fate of the mechanized universe, the materialist cosmology, which sees the material universe as the only reality, stripping it of soul.

A quote provided by Gary Lachman (2011), from *Book XI, Nous or Mind*, of the *Corpus Hermeticum*, succinctly presents many of the ideas included in this book regarding the importance of integrating the limited physical world and the unlimited unseen psychic world:

> Command your soul to go anywhere, and it will be there quicker than your command. Bid it to go to the ocean and again it is there at once. . . . Order it to fly up to heaven and it will need no wings . . . and if you wish to break through all this and to contemplate what is beyond, it is in your power. . . . If you do not make yourself equal to God you cannot understand him. Like is understood by like. Grow to immeasurable size. Be free from every body, transcend all time. Become eternity and thus you will understand God. Suppose nothing to be impossible for yourself. Consider yourself immortal and able to understand everything: all arts, sciences and the nature of every living creature. Become higher than all heights and lower than all depths. Sense as one within yourself the entire creation. . . . Conceive yourself to be in all places at the same time: in earth, in the sea, in heaven; that you are not yet born, that you are within the womb, that you are young, old, dead; that you are beyond death. Conceive all things at once: times, places, actions, qualities and quantities; then you can understand God. (as cited in Lachman, 2011, pp. 35–36)

Psychologist and astrologer Monika Wikman (2004), in her book *Pregnant Darkness*, suggested that spiritual practice is the way to achieving this sort of awareness of spiritual worlds living parallel to humans as they navigate through the physical manifestation into which they are born:

> How can we become unconscious again and again to drink from that deepest well of our being? Herein lies the heart of spiritual practice. In any spiritual tradition or lineage, dedication to a living practice is essential. Spiritual practice entails performing acts that assist us in dipping into, or immersing ourselves in, lunar consciousness, the unconscious, for renewal of consciousness. The shadow side of our modern spiritual eclecticism is that we risk not committing ourselves to spiritual practice, to daily dialogue with the numinous. Any technique that opens us to the irrational (for example, active imagination, meditation, dance, dreaming and dream work, chanting, drumming, yoga, exercise, sexuality, art, music), anything that helps us root in existence beyond the rational, has potential as spiritual practice. (p. xx)

Wikman suggested here a consistent practice to bring one to the unconscious depths of one's psyche—which also could be understood as the Egyptian *duat*, the underworld, the unconscious: One follows the Sungod on its journey, and then emerges on the other side into the light, the morning, of consciousness once again, only to repeat the cycle. Although the movement from one realm to the other suggests a duality, in reality, the realms are thought to reside together, as one, simultaneously. It is only the limitations of the physical world with its physical boundaries and laws of order that create an illusion of inaccessibility and the necessity of ritual to penetrate the self-created veil.

Many current writers, scholars, and analysts have made effort in their work and practice to integrate an awareness of ancient mythological and spiritual sensibilities.

During Jung's time several of the spiritual movements discussed in Chapter 6 were either already established or were just beginning to get a foothold—most notably Rudolf Steiner's Anthroposophy movement. In the foreword to *Jung and Steiner: The Birth of a New Psychology* (Wehr & Lauer, 2002), psychotherapist Robert Sardello (2002), cofounder of the School of Spiritual Psychology, wrote:

> We need Jung's psychology in order to remain imaginal. We need Steiner's spiritual science in order to apply this imagination to the forming of the world. These two together make possible a conscious, imaginal sun alongside the sun of our usual earthly consciousness. (p. 16)

Jung's imaginal psychology and its therapeutic technique is probably the most likely psychotherapy modality that incorporates the ancient Egyptian way of perceiving reality. Whereas most Jungian psychotherapy stays within the confines of the psyche and ventures out into the material world only as consequence and through the rather detached results of the therapy, Steiner's movement was intentionally in direct relation to the material physical world and was concerned with social and community development as well as individual accomplishment; in other words, it had conscious *material intention.* He did not, however, see the spiritual world and the material world as separate. To him, as with the ancient Egyptians, the material world was infused with spirit. This is an important distinction and should be duly noted. It can be argued that the whole purpose behind psychotherapy is to facilitate an individual's navigation through the material world, through relationship with others, community, and with the environment; however, Jungian depth psychotherapy focuses on the imaginal, inner world through dreams, active imagination, and unconscious complex processes. Sardello again illustrated this distinction:

> Jung always traces a symptom back to an archetypal image, looks for the gods or spirits or dead in the disease, and speaks always of such figures as images in the soul. Steiner looks at the same symptoms and also traces the symptom back to the gods, the spirits, or the dead, but he takes these spirits as directly acting on the human being. Without Jung's perspective, these acts by spiritual beings would be taken literally, as if they were just like earthly beings, except perhaps a little more shadowy. Without Steiner's perspective, on the other hand, the truth of the actual presence of spiritual beings is sidestepped. (p. 19)

It is difficult to say whether Jung would have been more of a practitioner in the spirit of Steiner's anthroposophy if he had not been held back by the stigma of being labeled a mystic. There is no evidence of Jung and Steiner ever having had a serious dialogue—let alone even meeting. Several references are made in Jung's *Collected Works* (1953–1979) regarding Steiner and anthroposophy, none of them very enlightening.

Since Jung's death in 1961, several scholars and analysts have linked depth psychology with the cosmology of the ancient Egyptians. Ancient Egypt has seemed to be a hot topic in Jungian circles for quite some time. Theodor Abt, a Jungian analyst and professor of agronomy and economic planning, has added a profound voice to the field of Egyptology and is an expert on the Egyptian *Amduat* or afterlife. In the book *Knowledge for the Afterlife*, Abt and co-author Erik Hornung (2003), an Egyptologist, described the Egyptian journey of the Sungod through the *duat*, the underworld, on its journey in the night to return the next morning rejuvenated and young again. Abt and Hornung provided a highly detailed account of this journey, covering every hour of this sacred passage, and included translations of the pyramid texts as well as numerous illustrations of tomb paintings depicting the journey. They suggested that this journey was not only that of the pharaoh at the time of his death but also the journey of every man and woman during various times of significant transformation in their lives; thus, this journey is the alchemical transformation of psyche and consciousness that all human beings can experience.

Again, Abt and Hornung's (2003) interpretation of Egyptian religious beliefs involves the more conventional theme of psychological transformation. The depth psychological stance has been not to see this journey as a series of literal transformations, as described in texts and in imagery and symbol found in Egyptian tomb paintings, but rather as a symbolic and metaphoric illustration of a psychological journey. Considering all that has been discussed in this book regarding the ancient Egyptians' concept of nonduality—the material world and the ethereal world being one—they may have had a more literal interpretation, without excluding the symbolic internal experience of this journey but also not separating it from a physical experience—the transformations were then psychophysical.

Continuing with other, more current, Jungian investigations into ancient Egyptian cosmology and how it may relate to modern psychotherapy, consider Andreas Schweizer's (1994/2010) book *The Sungod's Journey through the Netherworld*. Schweizer is concerned with the psychological transformation as symbolized by the ancient Egyptian Sungod journey through the *duat*. Schweizer, a practicing Jungian analyst who studied Egyptology with Hornung, made a pertinent point regarding the possible necessity of keeping this transformational journey symbolic through imagery and storytelling narrative and thus separate from the physical living experience:

> Comparing the structure of the Amduat to the psychology of common human experience, we may say that this unequivocal separation of the hereafter from the transitory world of the living symbolizes protection: on the psychological level, it is protection of the realm of the unconscious from infringements and abuses by the ego, which can lead to misuse of the objective psyche and its numinous images for a mere ego-purpose. If Egyptians hoped to be accepted among the blessed dead and even to be identified with the Great God after death, they were expected to devote their lives totally to the service of this god, who was also called the Great *Ba*-soul. In the Amduat, all the deities and blessed dead who dwell on the banks of the subterranean stream live through this god and for him. (p. 33)

This passage illustrates an important consideration regarding the concept of integrating the unseen world with the material physical world. In the view taken in this book, the dangers of the individual ego structure's probable demand to exercise full control over the inner psyche's power to manifest in physical reality is a problem found demonstrated throughout history as an acute abuse of personal power. It seems that the ancient Egyptian system of religion, including a large and powerful pantheon of gods and goddesses along with a very rich mythological tradition, ensures that the focus of power remains in the collective and not in the individual. The collective, in this context, refers to the divine pantheon as well as the physical world as it relates to and remains in harmony with the unseen world of spirit. Schweizer's research suggests that the system the Egyptians developed with regard to their rituals, hierarchy of power, and pantheon of gods supports keeping power in alignment with *ma'at*—the essence of inner and outer harmony.

Thom Cavalli is another Jungian analyst who has written extensively on alchemical transformation as it is depicted in ancient Egypt. One of his major books on this topic is *Embodying Osiris*, in which Cavalli (2010) used the ancient Egyptian Osiris and Isis myth of death and resurrection to illustrate his ideas about alchemical transformation and renewal through a symbolic death and rebirth. He viewed this myth as a representation of the whole of life, with its cyclic processes forever turning and churning and bringing forth creation, dissolution, and further creation. He observed that Osiris "possesses intimate knowledge of the cycle of life, death, and transcendence. Osiris is not an object of beauty but rather the process of beauty" (p. 66). Cavalli went on to say that the creative, inner, imaginal world is the source of the material world, not the other way around (p. 66). His text is highly relevant to the ideas presented in this book: Does the psychotherapist who is informed of these Egyptian spiritual principles become more effective in his or her work with patients? Cavalli stated that the task of making the darkness conscious "is precisely what the alchemists were willing to do and what today is the dirty job handed over to therapists" (p. 92). Although there is more to the Egyptian perspective of spirit and matter than bringing the unconscious to conscious light, any sort of integration of light and dark, spirit and matter, soul and body requires a transformation accomplished in the journey through the underworld and the integration of the physical life with the *duat*.

Most, if not all, practitioners in any form of Jungian psychology or depth psychology believe their work to be soul work. Although there may very well be a quite diverse perception of exactly what that is, a common ground could conceivably be set in defining soul as it has been roughly described in this book—the awareness and appreciation of the alternate reality to physical form. If Jungian psychology, or any form of spiritual and transcendent psychology, is soul psychology, then why do we need a new methodology grounded in an ancient Egyptian cosmology? Maybe we don't need something entirely new. Maybe through a deeper awareness of that cosmology we can give more credence, as a society and culture, to the prevailing forms of soul psychology and pull these aspects of current methodologies out of the materialist's dustbin.

If we perceive the human race to be suffering from the disease of soul suppression and repression, then certainly mass psychotherapy, with the intent of awakening the sleeping soul, would be in order. This perception very well may shed light on the truth, and psychotherapists who resonate with the concepts presented in this book could take it upon themselves to practice with this intention in mind—tending the soul of the world through the soul-care of its human inhabitants. But again, how can knowledge of the ancient Egyptian's view of reality assist in pursuing this intention? This question, among others, is addressed in the next chapter.

References

Abt, T., & Hornung, E. (2003). *Knowledge for the afterlife: The Egyptian Amduat—A quest for immortality*. Zurich, Switzerland: Living Human Heritage.

Cavalli, T. F. (2010). *Embodying Osiris: The secrets of alchemical integration.* Wheaton, IL: Theosophical.

Copenhaver, B. P. (Trans. & Ed.). (1992). *Hermetica: The Greek* Corpus Hermeticum *and the Latin* Asclepius *in a new English translation, with notes and introduction.* Cambridge, England: Cambridge University Press.

Freke, T., & Gandy, P. (2008). *The hermetica: The lost wisdom of the pharaohs.* New York, NY: Tarcher/Penguin.

Jung, C. G. (1953–1979). *The collected works of C. G. Jung* (H. Read, M. Fordham, G. Adler, & W. McGuire, Eds.) (R. F. C. Hull, Trans.) (20 vols.). Princeton, NJ: Princeton University Press.

Jung, C. G. (1963). *Memories, dreams, reflections* (A. Jaffé, Ed.) (R. Winston & C. Winston, Trans.). London, England: Collins. (Original work published 1961)

Jung, C. G. (1964). Archaic man. In H. Read, M. Fordham, G. Adler, & W. McGuire (Eds.), *The collected works of C. G. Jung* (R. F. C. Hull, Trans.) (Vol. 10, pp. 50–73). Princeton, NJ: Princeton University Press. (Original work published 1931)

Jung, C. G. (2009). *The red book: Liber novus* (S. Shamdasani, Ed.) (S. Shamdasani, M. Kyburz, & J. Peck, Trans.). New York, NY: Norton.

Lachman, G. (2010). *Jung the mystic: The esoteric dimensions of Carl Jung's life and teachings.* New York, NY: Tarcher/Penguin.

Lachman, G. (2011). *The quest for Hermes Trismegistus: From ancient Egypt to the modern world.* Edinburgh, Scotland: Floris Books.

Lindorff, D. P. (2004). *Pauli and Jung: The meeting of two great minds.* Wheaton, IL: Quest Books.

Miller, A. I. (2010). *137: Jung, Pauli, and the pursuit of a scientific obsession.* New York, NY: Norton.

Pauli, W., & Jung, C. G. (2001). *Atom and archetype: The Pauli/Jung letters, 1932–1958.* (C. A. Meier, Ed.). London, England: Routledge.

Salaman, C., van Oyen, D., Wharton, W. D., & Mahé, J.-P. (Trans.). (2001). *The way of Hermes.* London, England: Duckbacks.

Sardello, R. (2002). Foreword. In G. Wehr & H. E. Lauer, *Jung and Steiner: The birth of a new psychology* (pp. 7–32). Great Barrington, MA: Anthroposophic Press.

Schwaller de Lubicz, R. A. (1982). *Nature word* (D. Lawlor, Trans.). West Stockbridge, MA: Lindisfarne Press. (Original work published 1963)

Schwaller de Lubicz, R. A. (1985). *The Egyptian miracle: An introduction to the wisdom of the temple* (A. VandenBroeck & G. VandenBroeck, Trans.). New York, NY: Inner Traditions International. (Original work published 1963)

Schweizer, A. (2010). *The sungod's journey through the netherworld: Reading the ancient Egyptian Amduat* (D. Lorton, Ed.). Ithaca, NY: Cornell University Press. (Original work published 1994)

Wehr, G., & Lauer, H. E. (2002). *Jung and Steiner: The birth of a new psychology*. Great Barrington, MA: Anthroposophic Press.

Whitney, M. (Director/Producer), & Whitney, M. (Producer). (1986). *Matter of heart* [Motion picture]. USA: Horizon.

Wikman, M. (2004). *Pregnant darkness: Alchemy and the rebirth of consciousness*. Berwick, ME: Nicolas-Hays.

Zabriskie, B. (2004). Imagination as laboratory. *Journal of Analytical Psychology, 49*(2), 235–242. http://dx.doi.org/10.1111/j.1465-5922.2004.00455.x

8

PERSONAL INSIGHTS TO A MODERN PSYCHOTHERAPY GROUNDED IN THE PRINCIPLES OF SACRED SCIENCE

The purpose of investigating the cosmic worldview of the ancient Egyptians in this book is not to formulate a new methodology for modern psychotherapy but rather to encourage a better-informed community of psychotherapists practicing present-day soul-tending methods. Although in this ancient way of being lies a modern way of being that could benefit the world in unimaginable ways, it would be close to impossible to expect a practice to develop out of this knowledge that could more or less instantly change the world for the better simply through the practice of a newly formed methodology. The reparation of the soul or, more accurately, the new awakening of the sleeping awareness of soul requires a slow and deliberate process, which resonates, with little or no conflict, with a modern sensibility and understanding. Practicing ancient Egyptian ways in a modern world would not only be, in the long run, inefficient but also clearly uninspired and out of place for most.

Several accepted modalities in practice today provide effective ways to awaken this sleeping soul awareness. Jungian psychology is one method that can be effective in carrying out this intention. As briefly presented in this book, Carl Jung was very interested in pursuing a search for soul in his patients as well as in himself. He may have been a little resistant to carrying his work too far into the material realm as, for example, Rudolf Steiner did, but his intentions were similar to Steiner's: to make the world more conscious and lift the veil that would reveal untruths for what they actually are. However, it is all too common for any of these methods to fall into disrepute due to their seemingly unscientific approach to psychology and the human condition. It would seem imperative to relinquish the hold that modern materialism has on humanity and accept an approach to reality that is all encompassing—a reality that includes the material as well as the nonmaterial. This imperative seems to be more distant than it ever has been, yet it is surely a necessity before any form of psychotherapy will be capable of penetrating the prejudice that a materialist paradigm has created. We must move beyond an understanding of psyche and the universe that only entertains a material definition.

As a psychotherapist, I have found it necessary to change my own perceptions and worldview in order to integrate the perspectives I have addressed in this book and become more effective in my own style of soul work with patients. Along with the usual avenues of spiritual research and enlightenment, I have completed training and study in depth psychology at a doctoral level and have gained experience working with patients in my own private practice. I was also drawn to Egypt at an early age and have continued to feed that initial curiosity. I have visited Egypt twice and have had a myriad of experiences there. As presented in Chapter 1, the visit I made almost twenty years ago was with my late wife Janice and two close friends, Frank and his wife Tracey. Being in Egypt was an experience of the body—a body that feels the heat and the sensations of sun and sand and gathers visual impressions of stone, marble, and hieroglyphics. My presence there also involved an intellectual process, which attempted to reconcile the visceral input with logic and reason from a materialist viewpoint and, ultimately, from that limited perspective, came up with no reconciliation.

The basis of my calling to Egypt is a soul connection that I felt in touring this amazing land—an experience that I cannot adequately describe in words but that can more effectively be illustrated in art or music. The energy of the ancient Egyptians is still present in the sloping sand dunes of the desert and in the rock, quarried and chiseled by ancient hearts and hands. Although the medium through which the ancient Egyptians expressed their heartfelt awareness is, for the most part, no longer appropriate for a modern sensibility, the manifestation of their artifacts and the presentation of their cosmology through their extant texts is testimony to the deep and complex way they interfaced with, reconciled, and created their reality.

In writing this book, I have been called upon to refer to my own personal soul search. The statement, "One's approach to a subject affects what can be seen and learned" (Coppin & Nelson, 2005, p. 39), describes plainly my personal approach as an author. My goal has been to present a work that explores the unique worldview of the ancient Egyptians, their concept of a sacred and soulful science, and the manner in which much of modern humanity's materialist worldview differs in its form and function. Throughout this work, my own personal attitude, dreams, interests, experiences, passions, and perspectives have been revealed and integrated with the interpretation of texts relating to the topic. This unique and personal alchemical hermeneutic methodology (a term credited to Veronica Goodchild, 2012, by Robert Romanyshyn, 2007) was intended to result in an equally unique and individual perspective.

Robert Romanyshyn (2007), a prominent depth psychology author and teacher, described a research methodology that puts soul forward as an integral component of the process. He wrote, "Soul is not inside us. It is on the contrary our circumstance and vocation. It surrounds us, and we are called into the world, as we are called into our work, through this kind of epiphany" (p. 9). My interest in ancient Egypt called me to this work. Egypt herself, with her swirling history of magic, ancestors, rituals, and relics of an ancient desert culture, called me to her. Romanyshyn described researchers' soulful connection to their research as an inner calling that indicates a responsibility to listen to the ethereal voices within and around them. Perhaps the first murmurings of this call came in the dream I will describe shortly—a dream I experienced in my very early years. Maybe the calling came earlier than that, even possibly from a life previously lived.

This "soul in mind" (Romanyshyn, 2007, p. 4) paradigm of research fits comfortably with a study of ancient Egyptian cosmology, which perceives the physical realm and the inner, vaporous realm as one and the same world. With such comments as "Religion is about the responsibility we have as humans to become aware of the part we play in bringing to greater awareness the God-image in the psyche" (p. 22) and "A science of soul would be less about religion and more about the recovery of a religious sensibility in a world that has lost touch with the sacred" (p. 23), Romanyshyn demonstrated an awareness of the basic tenets of Egyptian religious cosmology as it is presented in this book. My desire has been therefore to incorporate in this writing a focus on presentation with soul in mind, as defined by Romanyshyn:

> To do research with soul in mind is to be attuned to the fact that in one's work one is already being claimed by an-other story, that one's work is already situated within a larger pattern, and that in one's work, one is in service to something other than oneself. Within an imaginal approach, that larger tale to which one is in service is the unfinished business in the soul of the work, which makes its claims upon a researcher through his or her complexes for the sake of continuing that work. This unfinished business in the soul of the work lingers, for a complex researcher, within the shadows of culture as the weight of history. (p. 83)

This present work then proceeds partly in service of the Egyptian gods themselves—influenced by them in order to facilitate the telling of the continuing story of ancient Egypt.

As mentioned in the preceding pages, my first experience of Egypt, or at least of something "Egypt-like," was a dream I had when I was 11 years old. The dream was not specifically about Egypt but had symbols and characteristics that, from that time on, I associated with the land of the Pharaohs. In the dream, I am a man of some authority—not a king, but possibly a king's aide or, more likely, a priest of some sort—in a land that seems to have the name of *Urn*. I am in a temple overseeing or simply observing some sort of ritual. It could be a burial or something equally important. A beautiful woman is involved in the dream but not present at the ritual. She comes in later, when I am back at either my place of residence or a different temple or sacred place. She hands me an object—a hand mirror or something of similar shape and size—which is bordered in a gilded frame. I take the object in my hand and walk out onto a terrace that overlooks a beautiful desert valley dotted with numerous structures, some with colorful flags flapping lazily in a diminutive desert breeze. I take a deep breath, taking it all in. Life is more wonderful than one could imagine, and as I wake up, I have a feeling of indescribable peace.

Although subjected to a fading memory, even today I feel there was not much more to the events of the dream than what is depicted in this account; however, it was not the events of the dream that held me captive for so many weeks, months, and even years after having it but rather the *feeling* that I had experienced. I had never had such a vivid dream—one that left me, after awakening, with the feeling that I had actually lived it rather than dreamed it.

I went to school that day and immediately told my best friend about the dream. Later that week, in my sixth-grade class, our Bible studies instructor (in the American south, in 1966, when Bible studies was still considered a valid part of the curriculum) passed around a book with a map of ancient biblical lands of the Middle East. (I have no recollection of the title of the book or its specific designated locations.) Caves were featured on the map (possibly the caves of the Dead Sea Scrolls), and as my best friend perused the book before it was passed to me, he suddenly looked up at me with wide-eyed excitement and said, "Look at the name of that cave, Todd!"

As the book was handed to me, I saw, in tiny print next to the black mouth of a small cave carved into the ancient cliffside, the word *Uri*—not quite *Urn* but close enough. I gasped, and a chill ran down my spine. I felt as if I had seen a ghost, and although, at the time, I knew nothing of Jung's (1952/1973 [*CW* 8]) theory of synchronicity, I felt, in the deepest part of my being, the significance of that moment. What it meant, I did not know, of course, and still do not know, except without that experience, this book probably would not have been written. This is a memory I have carried, supposedly intact, for 49 years. It was the feeling, the impact, and the realness of the dream and the subsequent discovery of the cave name *Uri* that captivated my young mind and soul then and continues to captivate me now. As I said earlier, there is nothing specifically Egyptian about the dream or the picture of ancient caves presented to me in my sixth-grade class, but throughout the rest of my life, I have always associated these experiences with Egypt and what I have come to know of this magical land.

So this was the beginning of my continuing call to Egypt, and this call has resulted in extensive study of the ancient Egyptian spiritual cosmology and then its integration with my other spiritual and psychological work throughout my life culminating with this book. For me, the call came early. I believe that, for many of us who practice some form of psychotherapy, the call does comes early, certainly not commonly in the form of dreams about Egypt, but in other imaginal and symbolic ways. I believe that the first step in developing a therapeutic style incorporating the concepts addressed in this book is to look within and nurture the soul-engaging events, both inner and outer, of a person's life—to put meaning and intention behind those events that were experienced and remembered as numinous and psychically powerful, and to reference them to our physical life on the outside.

From this developed focal point, a psychotherapist can then better facilitate his or her patients' own search into their soul-enriching life events.

This, again, may not appear radically different from any course of soul-work psychotherapy, but the subtle difference is evident in the attitude and intention of the practitioner as well as the patient. As Jung may have implied, the moon represented in his patient's psyche is the real moon, and the material moon is the illusion. Although it is not a requirement to see the physical world as illusion, the implication here is that it is neither more significant nor represents any more of a reality than the psychic world. When we begin to see this truly, and incorporate this insight into our paradigm of reality, we will begin to experience the inner and outer world as the ancient Egyptians experienced it and thus begin to experience an easy, effective, and creative flow between the two—as one.

My own psychotherapy practice has been influenced by my developing awareness of applying a concept of sacred science to my therapeutic work. I do not believe that this concept can simply be laid into my psyche and, as a result, radically change my perception of the world and reality and thus have a direct impact on my work with patients. Through my performance of ritual, meditation, and spiritual practice, however, I believe I have come to a greater understanding of how these mysterious forces penetrate what before seemed to be a dead reality. There is now more soul in my work, more consciousness of the heart, and more of an awareness of the dynamic powers present within the symbols, ideas, imaginations, and physical objects that come into my experience through my work with my psychotherapy patients.

One thing that I found difficult to ascertain in my research was the difference between the practice of archetypal and imaginal psychology, as Jung and his successors have described it, and a practice infused with spirit, as the ancient Egyptians may have defined it. As said above, I believe if there is a difference in the practice itself, it is a subtle difference, and lies more in the nuance of awareness and interface with the issues, images, and physical objects that come into the therapy container. How I practice psychotherapy now is different from how I practiced it previously, and it seems that the results for my patients are different. I seem to see and feel a living presence in everything that is presented. I am not only interested in the metaphor or direct meaning of symbol but am attuned to a living value to the symbol itself. Within that object, thought, imagination, or symbol is a rich life of detail and nuance. Not only is this an expansion of the thing known, but it is also utilized and becomes infused and integrated with the present experience, as if the present experience contains within it the whole of the past and the whole of future potential.

As presented earlier in this book, the thing itself that is entering into the transference field in therapy contains much more than its physical or even imaginal attributes. Bauval (1999) noted that the Egyptian hieroglyph described as *the wagtail bird* would not merely represent the wagtail itself but also everything that may be associated with the wagtail and the Egyptians' experience of it. He wrote, "The full knowledge of the appearance of the wagtail in Egypt should evoke the idea and the moods of the autumn equinox, the receding waters of the Nile, the rich soil of the valley, [and] the purity of the western deserts" (p. 51). In a therapeutic session, every symbol, idea, imagining, or physical object that presents itself likewise has such an expanded meaning, and although it is impossible to know the full extent of this meaning, it is possible to regard it, respect it, and honor it as entirely real and substantial.

The following practice dialogues are not transcriptions of actual events. They are instead composites of a number of therapeutic experiences with numerous clients as well as a mixture of imaginal and dream material intended to emulate a series of psychotherapy sessions engaged in this enhanced approach to my practice. None of the names presented implies or represents any real person or any real therapy session. If any of these events took place in actuality, they were only small suggestions that have been expanded upon through imagination and fictional narrative. These dialogues are examples of baby steps toward an expanded awareness and integration as described throughout this book. A person must learn to walk before running, therefore please be patient with the seeming simplicity of these accounts and insights.

Dialogue one

A new patient sat in the waiting room several minutes before his noon appointment. He was a young man, about 25 years old, with a full head of sandy hair and a pale, freckled complexion.

"Hi, Randy," I said as I stepped out of my office to greet him.

"Oh, hi," he replied, seeming a bit nervous.

I was aware of the dim lighting in the waiting room, and between our words of greeting, I could hear the ubiquitous burbling of the little Japanese fountain that Cindy, my wife and business partner, and I had installed in the room to mask or at least render unintelligible any possible leakage of conversation from either of our adjoining therapy offices. I asked Randy to come in my office.

As he was passing in front of me to enter the consulting room, something popped into my mind: a seemingly unrelated thought about a book I had been curious about earlier in the day. I wanted to see if Cindy had the book in her collection in her office. I knew it would take just a second to check, and I did not want to put it off, as I was certain to forget it as soon as the thought left my mind. Randy was my last patient that day, Cindy was not in the office, and I was sure I would be in a hurry to get home once my session was finished.

"I'll be right in, Randy, I just have to check something," I said politely, as I stepped into Cindy's office and shut the door. The book was there, although it took a few minutes of searching to find it. I pulled it from the shelf and put it under my arm to bring into my office so I would not forget it.

When I stepped into the other room, Randy was sitting on the edge of the couch, turned slightly to the right, staring intently at a print I have on the wall adjacent to the therapy couch. It is a print of Michael Parkes's painting, *Desert Dream* (see Figure 8.1). My office is filled with visually stimulating artifacts: a complete sandtray collection of figurines and small toys and objects used in

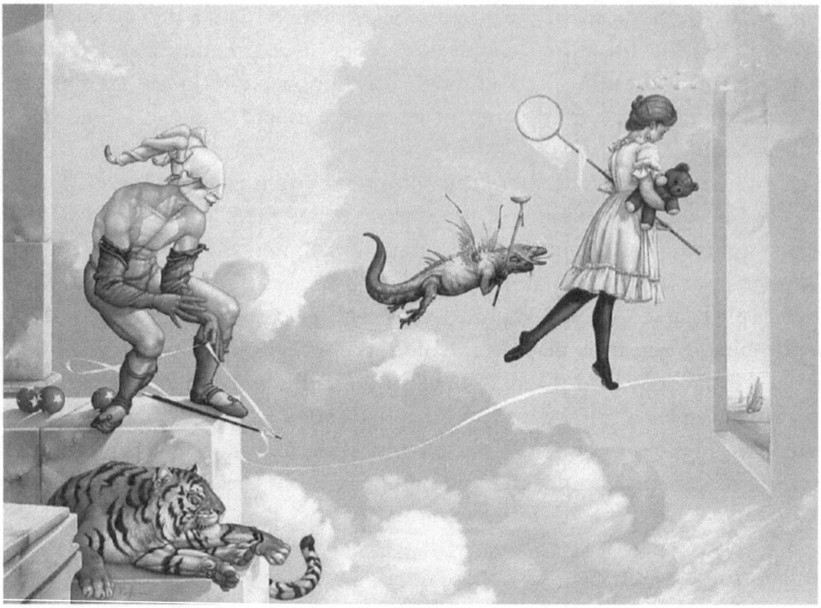

FIGURE 8.1 *Desert Dream*. Poster of painting by M. Parkes, 1986. Copyright by M. Parkes. Reprinted with permission.

sandtray therapy, many prints and photographs of evocative art, and other objects of interest I have collected over many years of travel to places such as Egypt, India, Malta, the American Southwest, and Russia.

In the past, I would possibly have asked Randy a cursory question regarding what he thought about the print. That day, however, I was moved by something that seemed to be occupying the room with us. I thought of Jung's (1946/1969 [*CW 16*]) diagram of the transference field (see Figure 8.2) and wondered from where in that field this energy was emanating. Could it be coming from outside the field—an objective reality beyond Randy and me—the collective unconscious? Or was it something else? I went with the flow and, deciding to follow my intuition, focused on the print and Randy's possible interest in it.

"What do you see, Randy?" I asked. Although I may have typically ventured down this route of inquiry as a depth psychologist, I was curious more about the print itself and what it was wanting to say to Randy rather than what Randy wanted to say about it.

"I don't know. It is rather interesting, though. What does it mean?"

"What do you think it means?" I replied, in classic therapist style. Randy continued to ponder. Finally, after several minutes went by, he said:

> The little girl is trying to follow her dreams, she has a net to collect them, and walks toward the opening into a new world, she walks on a ribbon, so her path is narrow and tenuous. The guy with the mask is her friend, trying to guide her.

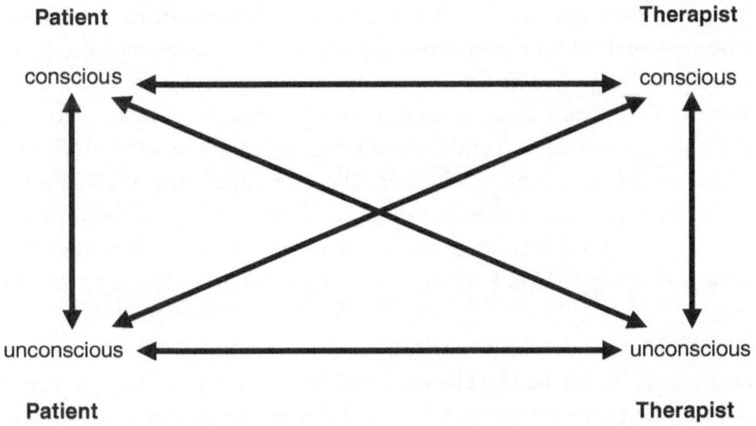

FIGURE 8.2 Jung's interactive field model. From "The Psychology of the Transference," by C. G. Jung, 1946/1969, p. 221. Copyright 1954 by Bollingen Foundation.

After this first dialogue encounter with Randy, several clients commented on this painting. It is interesting how everyone interpreted it differently. One woman saw the long-poled net the little girl was carrying as a spear or lance penetrating her heart through her back. Very few people have viewed the masked jester character as benevolent. Where is the objective reality in the symbols in this painting that draws from each of us such different feelings and associations? Many ideas flooded my mind at the time, including the importance of image as Hillman (1975, 1983, 2010) described it, Jung's (1952/1956, 1964) original theories on symbols, and depth psychologist James Hollis's (2000) ideas in *The Archetypal Imagination*. How did these conceptions differ from what Schwaller de Lubicz and others have said about Egyptian symbology or even about sacred science and consciousness of the heart?

Could depth psychology as it is practiced today still be hiding in the shadows, unwilling to step out into the consciousness of culture and admit that practicing a therapy with soul in mind necessitates a personal belief in the unseen nature and content of reality? Jung himself did not publically admit he was a mystic at heart (Lachman, 2010) and did not publically discuss his alleged belief that the pots and pans in his kitchen at Bollingen (Whitney & Whitney, 1986) had autonomous minds and intentions. Did he believe this himself?

Moving back to Parkes's painting (Figure 8.1), as I suggested, maybe in a modern context, this is indeed a demonstration of a fragment of the ancient Egyptian cosmology. Recognizing the painting's characters to be autonomous elements in our all-encompassing reality and seeing the painting, the room containing the painting, and each of us engaged in the therapy or, put better, the practice of understanding more deeply what it all means, is consciousness of the heart taking effect in the material world. The ancient Egyptians experienced a reality that would have been much easier to perceive as consensual than what we experience today. The richness of diversity in our modern day—diverse cultures, knowledge, symbols, technology, art, any sort of expression, and even nature and our physical environment—is far greater proportionally than what the ancient Egyptians had in their collective experience. The meanings and images we create in our minds that represent the autonomous energies that permeate the unseen reality around us could be just as varied in form and meaning as we are as individual, complex beings. The specific meaning we individually assess may not be as significant as the power the image holds to elicit change, understanding, and awareness in us.

Referring to his interpretation of the girl in the painting as following her dream, Randy finally muttered, "Am I right?" taking his gaze off of the print and looking back at me.

"I think so," I said.

As it turns out, Randy had had trouble finding his calling in life. At a very young age, he was pushed into accepting a responsibility in life that superseded in importance any desire or dream he may have harbored for his own path. He was frustrated with his job. He felt he was tied down to a way of life that was necessary to maintain his family's happiness and well-being. He had never followed his own dreams.

"What about the strange creature floating behind the little girl?" I asked.

Randy looked back at the picture.

"I don't really know," he finally said, after a moment of serious pondering. "Maybe that could be some example of serious threat to her, something she would have to face if she turned back."

I looked at the painting. I have often wondered about that creature myself. It has two heads; carries a strange contraption that holds a bowl of fire; and, most curiously, holds an egg in one of its back feet. I have always wondered about that egg and how this rather coarse creature is holding it so delicately with its thumb and forefinger—its pinky daintily held up, like a Victorian woman of the aristocracy would hold a delicate teacup. I was about to ask Randy what he thought of the egg but decided not to, as it seemed he had chosen to make no comment on his own about it and possibly had not even consciously noticed it.

The therapy with Randy ended after about eight weeks. It seemed to me to be good work, and most of it revolved around the print in my office. We often spoke of it and often asked of it certain questions, some obvious and some wherein neither one of us was clear on what was being asked. Randy commented once that he often wondered what would have happened if I had not needed to leave the room at the beginning of that first therapy session two months previous. I had often wondered that myself. What provoked me to feel the necessity to go into Cindy's office and look for that book? If I had not done so, I doubt if Randy ever would have noticed the print on the wall, and the therapy possibly would have gone in an entirely different direction, with possibly entirely different results.

Dialogue two

I have, on several occasions, for various reasons, told patients that I believed in fairies. Their response was usually laughter, assuming I was just being silly. I usually left it at that. One patient, a young adult woman I'll call Rebecca, who had, at a much earlier age, been diagnosed with borderline personality disorder, exclaimed happily, in response to my disclosure, "Oh, so do I, of course." I smiled.

"Literally?" I said.

"Oh, yes. I haven't actually seen any, but I do believe they exist and are out there somewhere."

I nodded my head. I wondered how I would have felt if Rebecca had said she actually had seen fairies. I told her that I agreed but had also never seen any. She was intrigued and curious.

"I thought that meant you were crazy. Magical thinking and all that, right?" she said.

Due to her long history of psychiatric care, Rebecca was familiar with the American Psychiatric Association's (APA, 2013) *Diagnostic and Statistical Manual of Mental Disorders* (*DSM-5*)—a clinical tome used by psychiatrists and other mental health care professionals to help ascertain specific mental illnesses and disorders.

"Yes, I suppose it does . . . mean I'm crazy," she concluded. I was not sure where I should go with this.

"Why do you believe in fairies?" I asked.

"Because it makes sense to me that they are real, and so does a lot of other things we are told are not real. I don't believe in *everything* mind you . . . just the stuff I am pretty certain of."

"And how do you know what you are certain of?" I asked, wondering about how I would answer the same question.

"I don't really know," she said. "I just feel it. It just makes sense."

I pondered on the difficulty of bringing an awareness of a spiritual world infused not only with spirit but also with actual *spirits* into the lives of the world's mostly rational and materialist human inhabitants. It seemed to me to be quite a tricky proposition. Maybe there actually are no fairies out there, but simply believing there are is enough. The belief in fairies, however, has to be more than a belief in little creatures that fly about in the forest. They have to have some sort of meaning, some sort of purpose in our everyday life, or, again, is it merely the *belief* in them that gives them meaning and purpose?

There are many accounts of terminal cancer patients who have imagined various sorts of creatures in their bodies fighting off the cancer and have been miraculously healed (O'Donnell, 2000; Siegel, 1986). Is this merely psychosomatic—a purely subjective and psychological phenomenon—or are there actually nonmaterial creatures, maybe not in the *form* that one imagines, but an autonomous, objective power that is engaged in the eradication of cancer? These are questions I certainly cannot answer, but they are, indeed, at the heart of the topic of this book. I think the best that I can hope for in my own practice is consciously to honor this awareness and consciousness that comes from the heart in my patients and in me. I have seen that this method has brought about positive results in my therapy with patients.

Rebecca was fragile in many ways, mostly due to the unconscious complexes that had formed at a very early age, being a child in a highly abusive family. Maybe her belief in fairies and other magical powers came about as a result of her psychological pathologies. Maybe, as the *DSM-5* (APA, 2013) would describe them, the visions were pathologies themselves. Conversely, perhaps her complexes were the wound that opened up the door to a deeper awareness of the imaginal world within—a world that also seeped out into the materialist realm of physical reality and became mixed into that realm just as watercolors blend on the artist's palette. Rebecca was highly creative and spent hours in her little studio creating stunning paintings on canvas and paper. Her artwork held within it an awareness of life and suffering impossible to put into words. In this world, she was happy, fulfilled, and found meaning. In the material world of work, relationships, and material survival, she was usually lost and suffered greatly. She believed her fairies were out there in that world, but they never could materialize because they did not follow the rules of materialism. Maybe, if Rebecca had lived in ancient Egypt and was open to this imaginal world without having to have been wounded, and had been accepted in the outer world as well as the inner, she would have actually seen her fairies.

A world where a consciousness of heart reigns as the spiritual paradigm and where soul permeates all that is experienced does not necessitate the existence of fairies or other magical creatures; however, it does allow for their appreciated influence and place in a person's whole awareness. A materialist, soulless paradigm limits the value of the unseen, imaginal world. What is the materialist value of a doctor who shares a bit of personal insight about a patient with his staff right before surgery (Denney, 2012)? Can the value of learning about a patient's interests, loves, and passions be measured? Can it be felt in a way that has positive consequences for the task at hand, the surgery about to be performed? Because its usefulness cannot be measured, this personal insight into a patient's life is of no value in today's practice of medicine. Only if there were a material benefit such as a measurable lessening of muscular tension, physical stress indicators, or the like, would it be considered beneficial. Since the patient is unconscious during this event, any positive effect could not enter the patient's awareness through the conscious senses. There is little to no material value recognized in honoring soul through nurturing of more intimate, human, connection with a patient in the reverie of the moment and the unseen affect of the group's participation in the event. This respect for soul does not necessarily have to involve the sharing of a patient's personal information; it could be in the form of a silent reverie, an appreciation, and an acknowledgment of greater things at work in a medical procedure than the movement of atoms.

This sort of awareness is, of course, practiced in many cultures through organized religion or deference to a personal form of spirituality. Many people practice this awareness in a personal way, through attention to dreams; faith in themselves and their fellow humans; and love of partners, children, family, and community. Rudolf Steiner's (1911, 1994, 1998) efforts with his anthroposophy are powerful examples of where consciousness of the heart could take us in a more modern setting. His community programs, agricultural programs, architecture, educational philosophies, and attitudes toward animals and the natural world were all evidence of a profound belief in the awareness of and interaction with soul. There have been other attempts to infuse soul into not only art and religion but also everyday life, community, and the sciences. It could be argued that all religions have this goal in mind to some extent, and although a considerable split has existed between science and religion, the practitioners of science and medicine can still find personal comfort in a belief system that includes a soulful perspective on life and the material world.

Both Randy and Rebecca, however, seem to be entirely unconcerned about this bigger picture. They live lives filled with inadequacies; minor and major sufferings; and dissatisfaction in work, relationships, economic fulfillment, and their personal quest for meaning. They do not see their problems as sprouting from a soulless world, soulless medicine and science, or even soulless religion. They see the problems, at least consciously, as mired in the inabilities and incapability of their partners to give them what they desire and the seemingly impossible task of finding work that is satisfying and brings in enough money to buy the things that bring them pleasure. They see the problems in their lives as attributable to the misunderstandings and callousness of their parents, their siblings, their partners, and their friends. If they go deeper in their personal therapy, they may find the problems rooted in an internal lack of self-esteem, a childhood that offered little love and much abuse, or other personal traumas that have rendered them helpless in dealing with life's challenges. If they go even further, maybe they will find a deeper disconnection with their soul and a disharmony with inner truth and the world of external experience.

Dialogue three

I once asked a patient, whom I will call Debbie, "What do you believe the meaning of your life to be?" She thought for a long while and finally said, "I don't know."

"What do you find really important to you in your life?" I asked—a smaller question.

"I don't know."

"What gives you pleasure . . ."

"I don't know," she interrupted, before I could finish my sentence. We sat in the silence for a moment. I could see the tension forming on Debbie's face. There was clearly frustration there. She could not even focus on what it was she wanted or found important. She did not seem to have ever addressed these core issues. Although Debbie's confusion is not the general rule with the patients I see, I do find it to be quite common.

Colin Wilson (1973), a contemporary English philosopher and novelist, wrote:

> The main trouble with human beings is their tendency to become engaged in the "triviality of everyday-ness" (to borrow Heidegger's phrase), in the suffocating world of their personal preoccupations. And every time they do this, they forget the immense world of broader significance that stretches

> around them. And since man needs a sense of meaning to release his hidden energies, this forgetfulness pushes him deeper into depression and boredom, the sense that nothing is worth the effort. (p. 5)

He also wrote:

> One day I believe man will have a sixth sense—a sense of the purpose of life, quite direct and un-inferred. This is Faculty-X. And the paradox is we already possess it to a large degree, but are unconscious of processing it. (front cover)

Both of these statements imply the sleepy nature of our awareness. Rebecca, Randy, and Debbie did seem to be asleep, suffocated by their world of personal preoccupations. Therapy, to some degree, did wake them up. For Randy, it was through a meaning he saw in Parkes's painting, a meaning he may see in many things with which he engages in his life, but such an abstract meaning, a nonmaterialist meaning, that usually he is afraid to express its importance. Rebecca was the same; the significance of fairies in her life, whatever detail that may involve, had no safe place to be until therapy. For Debbie, it was developing a greater awareness of the magical and wondrous life that swirled around her rather than a focus on the turbulence in her personal world and the incongruity in what she believed and what the prevailing, materialist culture told her to believe.

The ancient Egyptians seemed to have no difficulty in processing Wilson's (1973) Faculty-X. They had highly structured rituals, which, from a cursory analysis, seem much akin to Western religious rituals in Christianity, Islam, and Judaism. The core of their religious system, however, was internal. They appeared not to be suffocated by their personal preoccupations. This is an oversimplification of the obviously complex and dense Egyptian cosmology and practice, but from my own personal experience and observation, it does seem to be pertinent to this book.

What I have described here regarding my personal practice as a psychotherapist may not seem at all out of alignment with a practice committed to the methodology of depth psychology, transformative psychology, or even spiritual psychology. As I said previously, maybe a methodology thoroughly informed by ancient Egyptian sacred science, consciousness of the heart, symbology, and soul is not perceptibly different from the methodology pioneered by Jung and carried on today through the inspirations of Hillman, Hollis, Marion Woodman, and dozens of other practitioners and scholars in the field of archetypal and depth psychology. I do feel, however, that a nuance can be appreciated in this explication of Egyptian sacred science that may ultimately be at the heart of Jung's and even Hillman's (and possibly others') beliefs.

As mentioned earlier, these imaginal ventures into the reality of the inner world through personal psychotherapy are baby steps. However, to make this process of relating the inner world to the outer world a safe endeavor, it must be approached slowly and easily. There are many patients who are not nearly as open to this proposition as the three presented here. It is quite obvious this will not be a quick fix to the problems we may have encountered as a modern culture that has lost sight of soul through a limiting materialist paradigm. As psychotherapists we must first enlighten our own perspective of reality before hoping to pass that enlightenment to our patients, and when we do, we must be careful to avoid a directive through dogma. Our work is to facilitate a natural propensity we each possess that pushes us toward a consciousness, or intelligence, of the heart.

> We have borrowed the term "intelligence-of-the-heart" from the ancient Egyptians in order to designate that other aspect of man which allows us to penetrate beyond our animal limits and which, in truth, makes for human man's characteristic progression toward divine Man: the awakening of this original principle that lives dormant in every living human being. (Schwaller de Lubicz, 1960/1985, p. 12)

References

American Psychiatric Association. (2013). *Diagnostic and statistical manual of mental disorders* (5th ed.). Arlington, VA: Author.

Bauval, R. (1999). *Secret chamber: The quest for the hall of records*. London, England: Century.

Coppin, J., & Nelson, E. (2005). *The art of inquiry: A depth psychological perspective*. Putnam, CT: Spring.

Denney, M. (2012). *Nobody's boy: An old doctor and a new science* [Kindle DX version]. Retrieved from http://www.amazon.com/Nobodys-Boy-Doctor-Science-ebook

Goodchild, V. (2012). *Songlines of the soul: Pathways to a new vision for a new century*. Lake Worth, FL: Nicolas-Hays.

Hillman, J. (1975). *Re-visioning psychology*. New York, NY: Harper.

Hillman, J. (1983). *Archetypal psychology: A brief account—Together with a complete checklist of works*. Dallas, TX: Spring.

Hillman, J. (2010). *Alchemical psychology*. Putnam, CT: Spring.

Hollis, J. (2000). *The archetypal imagination*. College Station, TX: Texas A & M University Press.

Jung, C. G. (1956). Symbols of transformation. In H. Read, M. Fordham, G. Adler, & W. McGuire (Eds.), *The collected works of C. G. Jung* (R. F. C. Hull, Trans.) (Vol. 5). Princeton, NJ: Princeton University Press. (Original work published 1952)

Jung, C. G. (1964). Approaching the unconscious. In C. G. Jung & M.-L. von Franz (Eds.), *Man and his symbols* (pp. 18–103). Garden City, NY: Doubleday.

Jung, C. G. (1969). The psychology of the transference. In H. Read, M. Fordham, & G. Adler (Eds.), *The collected works of C. G. Jung* (R. F. C. Hull, Trans.) (Vol. 16, pp. 163–323). Princeton, NJ: Princeton University Press. (Original work published 1946)

Jung, C. G. (1973). Synchronicity: An acausal connecting principle. In H. Read, M. Fordham, & G. Adler (Eds.), *The collected works of C. G. Jung* (R. F. C. Hull, Trans.) (Vol. 8, pp. 417–531). Princeton, NJ: Princeton University Press. (Original work published 1952)

Lachman, G. (2010). *Jung the mystic: The esoteric dimensions of Carl Jung's life and teachings: A new biography*. New York, NY: Tarcher/Penguin.

O'Donnell, M. L. (2000). *Of monkeys and dragons: Freedom from the tyranny of disease*. San Antonio, TX: La Vida Press.

Romanyshyn, R. D. (2007). *The wounded researcher: Research with soul in mind*. New Orleans, LA: Spring Journal Books.

Schwaller de Lubicz, R. A. (1985). *Esoterism and symbol* (A. VandenBroeck & G. VandenBroeck, Trans.). New York, NY: Inner Traditions International. (Original work published 1960)

Siegel, B. S. (1986). *Love, medicine, and miracles: Lessons learned about self-healing from a surgeon's experience with exceptional patients*. New York, NY: Harper.

Steiner, R. (1911). *The education of children from the standpoint of theosophy* (M. Gysi, Ed.). Chicago, IL: Rajput Press.

Steiner, R. (1994). *Theosophy: An introduction to the spiritual processes in human life and in the cosmos*. Hudson, NY: Anthroposophic Press.

Steiner, R. (1998). *Art as spiritual activity: Rudolf Steiner's contribution to the visual arts* (M. Howard, Ed.). Hudson, NY: Anthroposophic Press.

Whitney, M. (Director/Producer), & Whitney, M. (Producer). (1986). *Matter of heart* [Motion picture]. USA: Horizon.

Wilson, C. (1973). *The occult: A history*. New York, NY: Vintage Books.

9

CONCLUSIONS

Several years ago, my late wife Janice and I took a trip to the Native American region of the United States in Colorado, New Mexico, Utah, and Arizona. The highlight of our trip was a visit to Chaco Canyon, a remote, limited-access archeological site in New Mexico that rivals Machu Picchu and similar, more famous sites in its richness of history and ancient architecture. Before visiting Chaco, we made a stop at the popular Mesa Verde region in Colorado, which is known for its Anasazi cliff dwellings. I have always been interested in the study of ancient cultures and found the trip to these sites to be intellectually as well as emotionally stimulating. Being a rather spiritual person, I was most interested in the more metaphysical aspects of these cultures and wanted very much to hear about their religious practices and more spiritual endeavors. What I experienced from the official word as it was conveyed by the trained rangers and tour guides was quite different from what I experienced in my gut, intuition, and even rational observation.

On visiting the Mesa Verde sites, I kept scratching my head after hearing the official talk on various aspects of life in the cliffs. Much of it did not make sense to me. Where were all of these people buried? It was explained that few remains had been found during excavations of the sites themselves (including the Pueblo Bonito site in Chaco Canyon) (Snow, 2010, p. 131). Why were the grain storage bins so small for such a large community? Why were there so many kivas (round rooms carved into the cliffs or built up from the ground), all deliberately built to exacting religious specifications? We were told that these were probably more commonly used as living quarters—but also were told that much of the Anasazi way of life was still a mystery. The same baffling explanations and speculations from the rangers accompanied our tours of the amazing excavations at Aztec Ruins and nearby Chaco Canyon, along with the insistence that the sites were built primarily as living communities where religious purpose was only a small part of the culture's activities.

I was reminded of the extant temple sites in Egypt, where one explanation for their continued existence after thousands of years was that they were built to last because they were temples. The ravages of the harsh desert had long ago consumed the everyday housing the community inhabited, as the care and attention required in the construction of a permanent structure was not a consideration. Needless to say, the rangers at these North American parks are supplied with small bits of information easily palatable to the general public who visit. I am not suggesting that more informed individuals and academics could not answer some of these questions more thoroughly, but why would the rangers present these queries as mysteries if there were easy answers available? I am no archeologist, and my puzzlement could be akin to the puzzlement a dog might experience looking at a skyscraper with no knowledge beyond ignorant speculation, but I was intrigued and decided to do more research regarding my questions.

My first bit of insight came from the popular American nature writer Craig Childs (2007), who implied in his book *House of Rain: Tracking a Vanishing Civilization across the American Southwest*, that my suspicions might be warranted. Although Childs never specifically stated that he believed the popular scientific conclusions to be incorrect, he did imply throughout his book that they might indeed be incomplete with regard to the early American Southwest cultures. His suppositions make sense, considering the dogma of scientism and the systematic abandonment of anything nonmaterial since Newton's time 400 years ago. As stated previously, it seems that, since that time, much of scientific inquiry has focused on a materialist reality and explanation for any mystery that may be found. The question arises: Could the description of this ancient culture's reality, as we see it in this modern time, possibly have been innocently manipulated in order to fit into the materialists' paradigm?

Materialism is a relatively new phenomenon in the world. In ancient times, when religion and spirituality took precedence over all other factors of life, wouldn't there have been more reason, say, for the Egyptians to have built the pyramids for purely spiritual and magical reasons than to have built them as a burial tomb for a king? Of the two choices, a burial chamber is quite a bit more practical and pragmatic, and that reason, therefore, fits more neatly into our current materialist worldview—considering there is very little, if any, evidence to support the burial chamber hypothesis. This book contends that the ancient Egyptians saw all science and all existence as sacred and that most endeavors in science, technology, and culture, in our modern materialist times, have lost their connection with soul. To be sure, the ancient architect–priests used a geometrical canon to design their monuments, but this canon was an intrinsic part of the sacred science of initiation. Geometry was sacred. Art was sacred. Architecture was sacred. Hieroglyphs were sacred. Astronomy was sacred. They were all part and parcel of a sacred science taught to high initiates in the temple. The mind of a human, which they deemed the most sacred thing of all creation, was to be made adept at this science or knowledge for the purpose of finding God.

As presented throughout this book, our culture's lost relationship to soul due to scientism and materialism probably touches nearly everything in our modern time. Even religion and spirituality, to a degree, has lost its connection to soul in the shadow of pragmatic materialism. Practicing a religion or spiritual discipline has, in many regards, become considered quaint and acceptable only because it is often excused as a fantasy or distraction rather than as a reliable belief system a person can depend on in their everyday life. Or, even worse, practicing a religion demonstrates a dysfunctional literalism found in the fundamental perceptions of that religion, which becomes a more destructive perspective than materialism.

Jung (1914/1961) seems to have suggested that it is a materialist's goal to reduce everything that we perceive in this world to a namable and identifiable element. I would go further to posit that the primary tenet of our current scientific worldview is to call *real* only those experiences that we can define in this limited manner. As mentioned before, the experiences that remain unnamed, unmeasured, and unpredictable fall into a category that contemporary philosophers have called promissory materialism (Tart, 2009), consisting of phenomena that will eventually be reduced down to their identifiable and thus definable parts within the current scientific definition of reality. This leaves a world and universe entirely defined by the cause-and-effect theory of Newtonian classical physics. B. Alan Wallace (2000), in *The Taboo of Subjectivity*, stated:

> Twentieth-century scientific materialism abandoned belief in any form of theism by adopting the principle of physicalism, which states that in reality only physical objects and processes exist. In other words, only configurations of space and of mass/energy and its functions, properties, and emergent epiphenomena are real. A closely related principle maintains that everything that exists is quantifiable, including the individual elements of physical reality, as well as the laws that govern their interactions. (p. 26)

Where does this limited view of reality leave the discoveries of quantum physics and noetic science? Apparently, nowhere at all. All experience that falls outside of the materialist view of the universe then becomes an intriguing mystery or colorful fantasy at best, and at worst, it is ignored. Returning to the alternative history point of view, not only are we not receiving the correct information (e.g., simply because it is considered impossible by the materialist scientists that the Egyptians could have built the pyramids using antigravity techniques or mind-over-matter metaphysics), but we also are missing a whole perspective of seeing reality, the material world, as a sacred place through integrating science with spirituality—thus creating a sacred science.

One might ask, "So what?" It is rather easy to use the idea of promissory materialism to put anything unexplainable on the back burner until material science catches up and provides explanations. Still, most people today do assume that Newton rules the universe, and nothing will come up that will defy these basic laws of physics such as the speed of light and cause and effect. Although quantum physics does seem to be challenging some of these laws successfully, according to most conventional physicists, quantum laws do not work the same way in the macro world, and therefore, we need not be bothered by them (Bohm, 1981; Goswami, 1997; Talbot, 1991).

Rudolf Steiner, as noted several times, made great efforts to change consciousness with his work in anthroposophy (Lachman, 2007), as have a myriad of other, more contemporary, spiritual efforts by various organizations; however, as I opened myself up to soul in my alchemical transference dialogue sessions, it was made clear to me again and again that the most efficacious process in this transition from a materialist focus to one of sacred science would be through the individual. An awareness of the sacredness and divinity in all things and all nonthings—a new paradigm that is not simply experienced as a dualistic concept of mind, body, and spirit but rather as an integrated whole—is only the beginning. As this new paradigm is integrated in the individual, possibly through a new perspective of psychotherapy, it will naturally move into the greater world of global awareness.

It seems evident that we now live largely in a world culture that has been dominated by the dogma of scientism—or a soulless science—and we are, as a whole culture and as individuals, not much better off for it. Depression is on the rise (Murray & Fortinberry, 2005), a general malaise seems to permeate the culture, and people seem to be more and more desperate to find meaning in their lives and grasp for a feeling of fulfillment and happiness while living them. In a truly mechanized universe, one never quite feels a master of one's fate. It all depends on where and at what speed the billiard ball hit the last ball—a universe of material cause and effect. Control is always local, with no feeling of any real power to change oneself, or the world, through thought or intention alone. With sacred science and soul restored to our material world, there is power and meaning in thought, love, awareness, imagination, and intention. Bernard Grad of McGill University conducted some experiments in the mid-1960s designed to demonstrate the power of healing (Tart, 2009, pp. 170–175). Although Grad was not the first or last to compile such data, his results were rather remarkable. Taking a number of laboratory mice, he deliberately wounded each mouse by cutting out a small piece of skin. Through a process careful to avoid typical pitfalls, he divided the mice into three groups: a control group, a group that received deliberate and conscious healing energy from a known human healer, and a group that simply received a treatment similar to the healing treatment (e.g., the same person holding the mouse in his or her hands in the same manner for the same amount of time) but with no intention to heal and not from a known healer. The difference in the rates of healing among the groups was quite extraordinary, with no materialist explanation for the higher rate in the second group. However, the second group had a controlled *intention* to heal, and therefore they were successful in their endeavor.

I do not propose that we make greater efforts to prove the scientific viability of these mindful, intentional, and soul-functioning phenomena. Although great strides have been made in the specific scientific experiments involving certain types of psi such as ESP, psychokinesis, and other similar phenomena (Radin, 1997), I do not personally believe that answers lie in simply defining these events in the same manner that we define most everything else in material existence.

Taking true advantage of what these phenomena can teach us or how they can help us see the world, the universe, life, and even material manifestation in a more expanded and more truthful manner will not come about through an objective, realist methodology. Achieving this new perspective thus becomes a matter of heart and not entirely intellect, and matters of the heart have not typically been viewed by science as empirically evidential. As this book has posited countless times, a truly fascinating aspect of the ancient Egyptians was their ability to manipulate the material world so effectively within what many have proposed to be a purely spiritual paradigm. As we have seen, they utilized the rules of material physics and mathematics, but it seems that they had at their disposal something much more.

As children, we are encouraged to fantasize, to bring elves and fairies to life, and to have imaginary friends and make-believe worlds; however, when a certain age is reached, and these nonphysical fascinations are continued, the young adult is considered mentally ill and needs treatment to bring him or her into the real world of quantifiable materialism. It is a shaky proposition to suggest, in our current limited mindset, that we all take fairies, ghosts, and even subjective feelings such as love, faith, and anything we would describe as numinous as seriously as we do cancer cells in our bodies, gold in the bank, and food on the table, but I believe that some effort must be made to find a place for these realities *as* realities and not merely epiphenomena of the chemistry in our brains. An argument could be made in favor of understanding an equality in our realities and thus not allowing the material reality always to be the most true. Our current Western cultural paradigm certainly would not grant this demotion or allow a smooth transition to this radical perspective, but our materialism may put much too much value on the physical life we hold so precious and thus block out other more meaningful and truthful awareness and value.

The current Western paradigm demands that individual experience be suspect until it becomes a group observation. Wallace (2000) commented on this condition:

> The principle of objectivism demands that science deals with empirical facts testable by empirical methods and verifiable by third-person means. This principle has proven to be very useful in revealing a wide range of facts that are equally accessible to all competent observers. Such facts must be public rather than private; that is to say, they must be accessible to more than one observer. However there are many other empirical facts—most obviously, our own subjective mental events—that are accessible only by first-person means and of which the only competent observer is oneself. (p. 22)

A thin veil exists between the subjective imagination and what is considered objectively real. I believe that our current culture and scientific paradigm demand that there be a distinction between these two realms of experience. Newtonian science, for the past 400 years, has provided a convenient measuring stick for this determination (Newton, 1962). There is hope, however, as presently our comfortable and delineated way of looking at the universe seems to be falling short. We are becoming more aware of the events that occur within our sphere of experience that fall outside the boundaries of causal science. Possibly, we are slowly going back to a sacred way of looking at reality, much in the same way the ancient Egyptians did. It seems in some ways to be a subtle shift, but the results of that shift, I believe, could be monumental in scope

Throughout this book, I have presented soul as being synonymous with a dynamic, unseen power alive in material things as well as the power of imagination, fantasy, and even the supernatural phenomena we occasionally encounter. It is difficult to describe what I mean by *soul*, and it may be best to leave it as an ineffable concept. My basis for describing soul in this way, again, comes from the sacred and spiritual paradigm in which many ancient cultures (including the pueblo people of Mesa Verde and Chaco Canyon) were ensconced. The principal tenet that can be gleaned from this book is that these cultures did not see a distinction between magic, religion, spirituality, the supernatural, Earth, the stars, animals, people, rocks, and temples and concepts such as mathematics or geometry. Everything in their lives was imbued with spirit and living spirits; everything was sacred and soulful.

Understanding, rather than just assimilating information, is a goal that few modern people seem to reach. The depression that afflicts individuals in our culture may be a result of confusion, frustration, and a feeling of being directionless. A sacred life is one of understanding, not in an intellectual sense, but in a heartfelt sense—a peace in knowing that not all can be known, yet it is always fruitful to seek answers. Understanding our purpose and meaning and knowing in our hearts that there is indeed meaning in the universe and in our lives—even though we may not be able to prove what that meaning is but simply know it is there—this, to me, is the nature of the sacred life: a life and a universe filled with soul. The ancient Egyptians seemed to understand this, and I believe that we can learn much more from them if we open our hearts and minds to their sacred way of being.

References

Bohm, D. (1981). *Wholeness and the implicate order*. London, England: Routledge.

Childs, C. (2007). *House of rain: Tracking a vanished civilization across the American Southwest*. New York, NY: Little.

Goswami, A. (1997). *Quantum mechanics* (2nd ed.). Dubuque, IA: Brown.

Jung, C. G. (1961). Some crucial points in psychoanalysis: A correspondence between Dr. Jung and Dr. Loÿ. In H. Read, M. Fordham, G. Adler, & W. McGuire (Eds.), *The collected works of C. G. Jung* (R. F. C. Hull, Trans.) (Vol. 4, pp. 251–289). Princeton, NJ: Princeton University Press. (Original work published 1914)

Lachman, G. (2007). *Rudolf Steiner: An introduction to his life and work*. New York, NY: Tarcher/Penguin.

Murray, B., & Fortinberry, A. (2005). *Raising an optimistic child: A proven plan for depression-proofing young children—for life*. New York, NY: Mcgraw-Hill.

Newton, I. (1962). *Sir Isaac Newton's mathematical principles of natural philosophy, and his system of the world*. Berkeley, CA: University of California Press.
Radin, D. I. (1997). *The conscious universe: The scientific truth of psychic phenomena*. New York, NY: HarperEdge.
Snow, D. (2010). *Archaeology of Native North America*. Boston, MA: Prentice Hall.
Talbot, M. (1991). *The holographic universe*. New York, NY: HarperCollins.
Tart, C. T. (2009). *The end of materialism: How evidence of the paranormal is bringing science and spirit together*. Oakland, CA: Noetic Books/New Harbinger.
Wallace, B. A. (2000). *The taboo of subjectivity: Toward a new science of consciousness*. New York, NY: Oxford University Press.

BIBLIOGRAPHY

Abraham, Hicks, E., & Hicks, J. (2007). *The law of attraction: The basics of the teachings of Abraham*. Carlsbad, CA: Hay House.

Abt, T., & Hornung, E. (2003). *Knowledge for the afterlife: The Egyptian Amduat—A quest for immortality*. Zurich, Switzerland: Living Human Heritage.

American Psychiatric Association. (2013). *Diagnostic and statistical manual of mental disorders* (5th ed.). Arlington, VA: Author.

Baigent, M. (2006). *The Jesus papers: Exposing the greatest cover-up in history*. San Francisco, CA: HarperSan Francisco.

Baker, M. C., & Goetz, S. (2011). *The soul hypothesis: Investigations into the existence of the soul*. New York, NY: Continuum.

Bard, K. A., with Shubert, S. B. (Eds.). (1999). *Encyclopedia of the archaeology of ancient Egypt*. London, England: Routledge.

Bauval, R. (1999). *Secret chamber: The quest for the hall of records*. London, England: Century.

Bauval, R. (2008). *The Egypt code*. New York, NY: Disinformation.

Bauval, R., & Brophy, T. G. (2011). *Black genesis: The prehistoric origins of ancient Egypt*. Rochester, VT: Bear.

Bauval, R., & Gilbert, A. (1994). *The Orion mystery: Unlocking the secrets of the pyramids*. New York, NY: Crown.

Bauval, R., & Osman, A. (2012). *Breaking the mirror of heaven: The conspiracy to supress the voice of ancient Egypt*. Rochester, VT: Bear.

Bernstein, J. (1989, February 27). A critic at large: Besso. *The New Yorker*, 86–94.

Bernstein, S. D. (1997). *Confessional subjects: Revelations of gender and power in Victorian literature and culture*. Chapel Hill, NC: University of North Carolina Press.

Blavatsky, H. (1965). *Isis unveiled*. Pasadena, CA: Theosophical University Press. (Original work published 1877)

Blavatsky, H. (1977). *The secret doctrine*. Pasadena, CA: Theosophical University Press. (Original work published 1888)

Blavatsky, H., & Codd, C. M. (1953). *The key to theosophy*. Adyar, Madras: Theosophical Pub. House.

Bleicher, J. (1980). *Contemporary hermeneutics: Hermeneutics as method, philosophy, and critique*. London, England: Routledge.

Bohm, D. (1981). *Wholeness and the implicate order*. London, England: Routledge.

Braden, C. (1987). *Spirits in rebellion: The rise and development of new thought*. Dallas, TX: Southern Methodist University Press.

Braude, S. E. (2007). *The gold leaf lady and other parapsychological investigations*. Chicago, IL: University of Chicago Press.

Brier, B., & Hobbs, A. H. (1999). *Daily life of the ancient Egyptians*. Westport, CT: Greenwood Press.

Budge, E. A. W. (1899a). *Egyptian magic*. London, England: Paul.

Budge, E. A. W. (Trans.). (1899b). *The book of the dead: The papyrus of Ani in the British Museum*. London, England: British Museum/Longmans.

Budge, E. A. W. (1989). *The Rosetta Stone*. New York, NY: Dover.

Burleigh, N. (2007). *Mirage: Napoleon's scientists and the unveiling of Egypt*. New York, NY: Harper.

Byrne, R. (2006). *The secret*. New York, NY: Atria Books.

Cambray, J. (2009). *Synchronicity: Nature and psyche in an interconnected universe*. College Station, TX: Texas A & M University Press.

Cartledge, P. (1999). *Democritus*. New York, NY: Routledge.

Castaneda, C. (1972). *Journey to Ixtlan: The lessons of don Juan*. New York, NY: Simon.

Cavalli, T. F. (2010). *Embodying Osiris: The secrets of alchemical integration*. Wheaton, IL: Theosophical.

Childs, C. (2007). *House of rain: Tracking a vanished civilization across the American Southwest*. New York, NY: Little.

Clark, R. (2000). *The sacred tradition in ancient Egypt: The esoteric wisdom revealed*. St. Paul, MN: Llewellyn.

Clark, R. (2003). *The sacred magic of ancient Egypt: The spiritual practice restored*. St. Paul, MN: Llewellyn.

Copenhaver, B. P. (Trans. & Ed.). (1992). *Hermetica: The Greek* Corpus Hermeticum *and the Latin* Asclepius *in a new English translation, with notes and introduction*. Cambridge, England: Cambridge University Press.

Coppin, J., & Nelson, E. (2005). *The art of inquiry: A depth psychological perspective*. Putnam, CT: Spring.

Corbin, H. (1998). *Alone with the alone: Creative imagination in the Sufism of Ibn Arabi* (R. Manheim, Trans.). Princeton, NJ: Princeton University Press. (Original work published 1958)

Cott, J., with El Zeini, H. (1989). *The search for Omm Sety: A story of eternal love*. Garden City, NY: Doubleday.

Courbin, P. (1988). *What is archaeology? An essay on the nature of archaeological research*. Chicago, IL: University of Chicago Press.

Cousineau, P. (1994). *Soul: An archaeology—Readings from Socrates to Ray Charles*. San Francisco, CA: HarperSanFrancisco.

Davies, P. C. W., & Gribbin, J. (2007). *The matter myth: Dramatic discoveries that challenge our understanding of physical reality*. New York, NY: Simon.

Denney, M. (2001). *Body, soul, and medicine: Confessions of an elder physician* (Doctoral dissertation). Available from Proquest Dissertations and Theses database. (UMI No. 3029756)

Denney, M. (2012). *Nobody's boy: An old doctor and a new science* [Kindle DX version]. Retrieved from http://www.amazon.com/Nobodys-Boy-Doctor-Science-ebook

Deutsch, D. (1997). *The fabric of reality: The science of parallel universes and its implications*. New York: Penguin Books.

Deutsch, D. (2001). In T. Folger, Quantum shmantum. *Discover, 22*:37–43.

Dodson, A. (1999). Carter, Howard. In K. A. Bard, with S. B. Shubert (Eds.), *Encyclopedia of the archaeology of ancient Egypt* (pp. 190–191). London, England: Routledge.

Dossey, L. (1993). *Healing words: The power of prayer and the practice of medicine*. San Francisco, CA: HarperSanFrancisco.

Doucet, C. (1990). *The Gospel according to Mary Magdalene*. Windsor, ON: Black Moss Press.

Drower, M. S. (1985). *Flinders Petrie: A life in archaeology*. London, England: Gollancz.

Dubois, G. (2006). *Fulcanelli and the alchemical revival: The man behind the mystery of the cathedrals*. Rochester, VT: Destiny Books.

Dunn, C. (1998). *The Giza power plant: Technologies of ancient Egypt*. Santa Fe, NM: Bear.

Dunn, C. (2008, July 1). Mega saws of the pyramid builders. *Atlantis Rising*, 32–65.

Einstein, A. (1961). *Relativity: The special and the general theory; a popular exposition*. New York, NY: Crown.

Eisenbud, J. (1989). *The world of Ted Serios: "Thoughtographic" studies of an extraordinary mind*. Jefferson, NC: McFarland.

Emerson, R. W. (1944). *The essays of Ralph Waldo Emerson*. New York: Barnes.

Everett III, H. (1957). "Relative state" formulation of quantum mechanics. *Reviews of Modern Physics, 29*, 454–462. See a digital version at: http://www.univer.omsk.su/omsk/Sci/Everett/paper1957.htm

Fillmore, C. (1947). *Christian healing: The science of being*. Kansas City, MO: Unity School of Christianity.

Finklestone, J. (1996). *Anwar Sadat: Visionary who dared*. London, England: Cass.

Flanagan, O. J. (2003). *The problem of the soul: Two visions of mind and how to reconcile them*. New York, NY: BasicBooks.

Folger, T. (2001). Quantum shmantum. *Discover, 22*(9), 37–43.

Franz, M.-L. von. (1980). *Alchemy: An introduction to the symbolism and the psychology*. Toronto, ON: Inner City Books.

Franz, M.-L. von. (1992). *Psyche and matter*. Boston, MA: Shambhala.

Freke, T., & Gandy, P. (2008). *The hermetica: The lost wisdom of the pharaohs*. New York, NY: Tarcher/Penguin.

Friedman, N. (1994) *Bridging science and spirit: Common elements in David Bohm's physics, the perennial philosophy and Seth*. St. Louis, MO: Moment Point Press.

Furlong, M. (1996). *Visions and longings: Medieval women mystics*. Boston, MA: Shambhala.

Gadamer, H. (1998). *Truth and method* (J. Weinsheimer & D. Marshall, Trans). New York, NY: Continuum. (Original work published 1960)

Goetz, S., & Taliaferro, C. (2011). *A brief history of the soul*. Malden, MA: Wiley-Blackwell.

Goodchild, V. (2012). *Songlines of the soul: Pathways to a new vision for a new century*. Lake Worth, FL: Nicolas-Hays.

Goswami, A. (1997). *Quantum mechanics* (2nd ed.). Dubuque, IA: Brown

Goswami, A. (2004). *The quantum doctor: A quantum physicist explains the healing power of integral medicine*. Charlottesville, VA: Hampton Roads.

Goswami, A., Reed, R. E., & Goswami, M. (1993). *The self-aware universe: How consciousness creates the material world*. New York, NY: Putnam.

Hamilton, B. (2003). *Religion in the medieval West* (2nd ed.). New York, NY: Oxford University Press.

Hancock, G., & Bauval, R. (1996). *The message of the Sphinx: A quest for the hidden legacy of mankind*. New York, NY: Crown.

Harmless, W. (2008). *Mystics*. New York, NY: Oxford University Press.

Hayen, T. M. (2003). On the very edge of magnificence. Unpublished manuscript.

Hayen, T. M. (2010). Logbook: Transference dialogues. Unpublished manuscript.

Heisenberg, W. (1990). *Physics and Philosophy*. London: Penguin. (Original work published 1962)

Herodotus. (2008). *The histories* (R. Waterfield, Trans.) (C. Dewald, Comment.). New York, NY: Oxford University Press.

Hillman, J. (1975). *Re-visioning psychology*. New York, NY: Harper.

Hillman, J. (1983a). *Archetypal psychology: A brief account: Together with a complete checklist of works*. Dallas, TX: Spring.

Hillman, J. (1983b). *Healing fiction*. Barrytown, NY: Station Hill Press.

Hillman, J. (1989). *A blue fire: Selected writings* (T. Moore, Ed.). New York, NY: Harper.

Hillman, J. (1996). *The soul's code: In search of character and calling*. New York, NY: Random House.

Hillman, J. (2010). *Alchemical psychology*. Putnam, CT: Spring.

Hollis, J. (2000). *The archetypal imagination*. College Station, TX: Texas A & M University Press.

Holmes, E. (1991). *Living the science of mind*. Marina del Rey, CA: DeVorss.

Holmes, E. (1997). *The science of mind*. New York, NY: Putnam.

Holmes, E., & Lathem, M. A. (1938). *The science of mind* (Completely revised and enlarged ed.). New York, NY: McBride.

Holmes, R. (2010). *The age of wonder: How the romantic generation discovered the beauty and terror of science*. New York, NY: Vintage Books.

Holmyard, E. J. (1990). *Alchemy*. New York, NY: Dover.

Husserl, E. (1975). *Experience and judgment: Investigations in a genealogy of logic* (L. Landgrebe, Ed.) (J. S. Churchill & K. Ameriks, Trans.). Evanston, IL: Northwestern University Press. (Original work published 1939)

Husserl, E. (2012). *Ideas: General introduction to pure phenomenology* (W. R. B. Gibson, Trans.). London, England: Routledge. (Original work published 1913)

Jones, W. T. (1975). *A history of Western philosophy, Vol. 5: The twentieth century to Wittgenstein and Sartre*. San Francisco, CA: Harcourt.

Judge, W. Q. (1951). *Practical occultism: From the private letters of William Q. Judge*. Pasadena, CA: Theosophical University Press.

Jung, C. G. (1953–1979). *The collected works of C. G. Jung* (H. Read, M. Fordham, G. Adler, & W. McGuire, Eds.) (R. F. C. Hull, Trans.) (20 vols.). Princeton, NJ: Princeton University Press.

Jung, C. G. (1956). *Symbols of transformation*. In H. Read, M. Fordham, G. Adler, & W. McGuire (Eds.), *The collected works of C. G. Jung* (R. F. C. Hull, Trans.) (Vol. 5). Princeton, NJ: Princeton University Press. (Original work published 1952)

Jung, C. G. (1961). *Some crucial points in psychoanalysis: A correspondence between Dr. Jung and Dr. Loÿ*. In H. Read, M. Fordham, G. Adler, & W. McGuire (Eds.), *The collected works of C. G. Jung* (R. F. C. Hull, Trans.) (Vol. 4, pp. 251–289). Princeton, NJ: Princeton University Press. (Original work published 1914)

Jung, C. G. (1963). *Memories, dreams, reflections* (A. Jaffé, Ed.) (R. Winston & C. Winston, Trans.). London, England: Collins. (Original work published 1961)

Jung, C. G. (1964a). Approaching the unconscious. In C. G. Jung & M.-L. von Franz (Eds.). *Man and his symbols* (pp. 18–103). Garden City, NY: Doubleday.

Jung, C. G. (1964b). Archaic man. In H. Read, M. Fordham, G. Adler, & W. McGuire (Eds.), *The collected works of C. G. Jung* (R. F. C. Hull, Trans.) (Vol. 10, pp. 50–73). Princeton, NJ: Princeton University Press. (Original work published 1931)

Jung, C. G. (1966). The aims of psychotherapy. In H. Read, M. Fordham, G. Adler, & W. McGuire (Eds.), *The collected works of C. G. Jung* (R. F. C. Hull, Trans.) (Vol. 16, pp. 35–52). Princeton, NJ: Princeton University Press. (Original work published 1929)

Jung, C. G. (1969). The psychology of the transference. In H. Read, M. Fordham, & G. Adler (Eds.), *The collected works of C. G. Jung* (R. F. C. Hull, Trans.) (Vol. 16, pp. 163–323). Princeton, NJ: Princeton University Press. (Original work published 1946)

Jung, C. G. (1970). Mysterium coniunctionis. In H. Read, M. Fordham, G. Adler, & W. McGuire (Eds.), *The collected works of C. G. Jung* (R. F. C. Hull, Trans.) (Vol. 14). Princeton, NJ: Princeton University Press. (Original work published 1955–1956)

Jung, C. G. (1973). Synchronicity: An acausal connecting principle. In H. Read, M. Fordham, & G. Adler (Eds.), *The collected works of C. G. Jung* (R. F. C. Hull, Trans.) (Vol. 8, pp. 417–531). Princeton, NJ: Princeton University Press. (Original work published 1952)

Jung, C. G. (2009). *The red book: Liber novus* (S. Shamdasani, Ed.) (S. Shamdasani, M. Kyburz, & J. Peck, Trans.). New York, NY: Norton.

Koch, T. (1995). Implementation of a hermeneutic inquiry in nursing: Philosophy, rigor and representation. *Journal of Advanced Nursing, 21*, 827–836.

Kragh, H. (1999). *Quantum generations: A history of physics in the twentieth century*. Princeton, NJ: Princeton University Press.

Kvale, S. (1996). *InterViews: An introduction to qualitative research*. Thousand Oaks, CA: Sage.

Lachman, Gary (2000, January–February). Rene Schwaller de Lubicz and the Intelligence of the Heart. *Quest, 89*(1), 4–11. Retrieved from https://www.theosophical.org/publications/quest-magazine/42-publications/quest-magazine/1281-rene-schwaller-de-lubicz-and-the-intelligence-of-the-heart

Lachman, G. (2006). *In search of P. D. Ouspensky: The genius in the shadow of Gurdjieff* (2nd ed.). Wheaton, IL: Quest Books.

Lachman, G. (2007). *Rudolf Steiner: An introduction to his life and work*. New York, NY: Tarcher/Penguin.

Lachman, G. (2010). *Jung the mystic: The esoteric dimensions of Carl Jung's life and teachings*. New York, NY: Tarcher/Penguin.

Lachman, G. (2011). *The quest for Hermes Trismegistus: From ancient Egypt to the modern world*. Edinburgh, Scotland: Floris Books.

Lachman, G. (2012). *Madame Blavatsky: The mother of modern spirituality*. New York, NY: Tarcher/Penguin.

Laverty, S. M. (2003). Hermeneutic phenomenology and phenomenology: A comparison of historical and methodological considerations. *International Journal of Qualitative Methods, 2*(3), 21–35.

Le Plongeon, A. (1983). *The origin of the Egyptians*. Los Angeles, CA: Philosophical Research Society.

Lehner, M. (1997). *The complete pyramids*. New York, NY: Thames.

Lehner, M., & Cayce, E. (1974). *The Egyptian heritage: Based on the Edgar Cayce readings*. Virginia Beach, VA: A.R.E. Press.

Lehner, M., Wetterstrom, W., Giza Plateau Mapping Project, & Ancient Egypt Research Associates. (2007). *Giza reports: The Giza Plateau Mapping Project*. Boston, MA: Ancient Egypt Research Associates.

Lin, Y. (1943). *Between tears and laughter*. New York: Day

Linden, S. J. (2003). *The alchemy reader: From Hermes Trismegistus to Isaac Newton*. Cambridge, UK: Cambridge University Press.

Lindorff, D. P. (2004). *Pauli and Jung: The meeting of two great minds*. Wheaton, IL: Quest Books.

Macaulay, D. (1975). *Pyramid*. Boston, MA: Houghton.

Malkowski, E. F. (2006). *Before the pharaohs: Egypt's mysterious prehistory*. Rochester, VT: Bear.

Malkowski, E. F. (2007). *The spiritual technology of ancient Egypt: Sacred science and the mystery of consciousness*. Rochester, VT: Inner Traditions.

Malkowski, E. F. (2010). *Ancient Egypt 39,000 BCE: The history, technology, and philosophy of Civilization X*. Rochester, VT: Bear.

Mansfield, V. (1995). *Synchronicity, science, and soul-making: Understanding Jungian synchronicity through physics, Buddhism, and philosophy*. Chicago, IL: Open Court.

Margolis, J. (2004). *O: The intimate history of the orgasm*. New York, NY: Grove Press.

Marshall, I. N., Zohar, D., & Peat, F. D. (1997). *Who's afraid of Schrödinger's cat? All the new science ideas you need to keep up with the new thinking*. New York, NY: Morrow.

Maspero, G. (1912). *Art in Egypt* (E. Lee, Trans.). New York, NY: Scribner's.

Matt, D. C. (1995). *The essential Kabbalah: The heart of Jewish mysticism*. San Francisco, CA: HarperSanFrancisco.

Maxwell-Stuart, P. G. (2008). *The chemical choir*. London, England: Continuum.

McClure, R., & Heffron, J. (2009). *Coral Castle: The mystery of Ed Leedskalnin and his American Stonehenge*. Columbus, OH: Ternary.

Mercatante, A. S., & Bianchi, R. S. (1995). *Who's who in Egyptian mythology*. Lanham, MD: Scarecrow Press.

Michelet, J., & Allinson, A. R. (1992). *Satanism and witchcraft: The classic study of medieval superstition*. New York, NY: Carol.

Miller, A. I. (2010). *137: Jung, Pauli, and the pursuit of a scientific obsession*. New York, NY: Norton.

Mishlove, J. (2000). *The PK man: A true story of mind over matter*. Charlottesville, VA: Hampton Roads.

Moran, D. (2012). Foreword. In E. Husserl, *Ideas: General introduction to pure phenomenology* (W. R. B. Gibson, Trans.) (pp. xiii–xxxiii). London, England: Routledge.

Murray, B., & Fortinberry, A. (2005). *Raising an optimistic child: A proven plan for depression-proofing young children—for life*. New York, NY: Mcgraw-Hill.

Napoleon and the Great Pyramid: Myth and reality. (2014). Retrieved from http://www.strangehistory.net/2013/12/02/napoleon-and-the-great-pyramid/

Napoleon I, E. o. t. F., Jomard, M., Lelorgne de Savigny, M. J. C. s., & Fourier, J. B. J. b. (1809–1829). *Description de l'Egypte: Ou recueil des observations et des recherches qui ont* été *faites en Égypte pendant l'expédition de l'armée française* [Description of Egypt, or the collection of observations and research which were made in Egypt during the expedition of the French Army] (23 vols.). Paris, France: Impériale.

Napoleon's visit to the Great Pyramid. (2014). Retrieved from http://www.gizapyramid.com/history.htm

Naydler, J. (1994). *On the divinity of the Gods*. Oxford, England: Abzu.

Naydler, J. (1996). *Temple of the cosmos: The ancient Egyptian experience of the sacred*. Rochester, VT: Inner Traditions.

Naydler, J. (2005). *Shamanic wisdom in the pyramid texts: The mystical tradition of ancient Egypt*. Rochester, VT: Inner Traditions.

Naydler, J. (2009). *The future of the ancient world: Essays on the history of consciousness*. Rochester, VT: Inner Traditions.

Newton, I. (1962). *Sir Isaac Newton's mathematical principles of natural philosophy, and his system of the world*. Berkeley, CA: University of California Press.

Newton, I. (1995). *The principia*. Amherst, NY: Prometheus Books.

O'Donnell, M. L. (2000). *Of monkeys and dragons: Freedom from the tyranny of disease*. San Antonio, TX: La Vida Press.

Palmer, R. (1969). *Hermeneutics: Interpretation theory in Schleiermacher, Dilthey, Heidegger, and Gadamer*. Evanston, IL: Northwestern University Press.

Parker, J. (2011). *The soul solution: Enlightening meditations for resolving life's problems*. Tiburon, CA: Kramer/New World Library.

Pauli, W., & Jung, C. G. (2001). *Atom and archetype: The Pauli/Jung letters, 1932–1958*. (C. A. Meier, Ed.). London, England: Routledge.

Peat, F. D. (1987). *Synchronicity: The bridge between matter and mind*. New York, NY: Bantam Books.

Picknett, L. (2003). *Mary Magdalene: Christianity's hidden goddess*. London, England: Robinson.

Picknett, L., & Prince, C. (2011). *The forbidden universe*. London, England: Constable.

Polkinghorne, D. (1983). *Methodology for the human sciences: Systems of inquiry*. Albany: State University of New York Press.

Popper, K. (1958, Summer). The representation of nature in contemporary physics. *Daedalus 87*, 95–108.

Porter, R. (2001). *The Enlightenment* (2nd ed.). New York, NY: Palgrave.

Pregadio, F. (2006). *Great clarity: Daoism and alchemy in early medieval China*. Stanford, CA: Stanford University Press.

Quimby, P. (1921). *The Quimby manuscripts* (H. Dresser, Ed.). New York, NY: Crowell.

Radin, D. I. (1997). *The conscious universe: The scientific truth of psychic phenomena*. New York, NY: HarperEdge.

Ray, J. (2007). *The Rosetta Stone and the rebirth of Ancient Egypt*. London, England: Profile.

Rock, A. (2005). *The mind at night: The new science of how and why we dream*. New York, NY: Basic Books.

Romanyshyn, R. D. (2007). *The wounded researcher: Research with soul in mind*. New Orleans, LA: Spring Journal Books.

Romer, J. (2012). *A history of ancient Egypt: From the first farmers to the Great Pyramid*. London; New York, NY: Allen Lane.

Rosenblum, B., & Kuttner, F. (2011). *Quantum enigma: Physics encounters consciousness*. Oxford, England: Oxford University Press.

Ryan, C. J. (1911). The new Egyptology and the theosophical records. *Theosophical Path, 1*(1), 15–19.

Ryan, C. J. (1939). *What is theosophy? A general view for inquirers*. Point Loma, CA: Theosophical University Press.

Sacred. (2011). In *Oxford advanced American dictionary*. Retrieved from http://oaadonline.oxfordlearnersdictionaries.com/dictionary/sacred

Salaman, C., van Oyen, D., Wharton, W. D., & Mahé, J.-P. (Trans.). (2001). *The way of Hermes*. London, England: Duckbacks.

Sardello, R. (2002). Foreword. In G. Wehr & H. E. Lauer, *Jung and Steiner: The birth of a new psychology* (pp. 7–32). Great Barrington, MA: Anthroposophic Press.

Schoch, R. M. (2012). *Forgotten civilization: The role of solar outbursts in our past and future*. Rochester, VT: Inner Traditions.

Schoch, R. M., with McNally, R. A. (1999). *Voices of the rocks: A scientist looks at catastrophes and ancient civilizations*. New York, NY: Harmony Books.

Schoch, R. M., & McNally, R. A. (2005). *Pyramid quest: Secrets of the Great Pyramid and the dawn of civilization*. New York, NY: Tarcher/Penguin.

Schwaller de Lubicz, R. A. (1978). *Symbol and symbolism* (D. Lawlor & R. Lawlor, Trans.). New York, NY: Autumn Press. (Original work published 1951)

Schwaller de Lubicz, R. A. (1982). *Nature word* (D. Lawlor, Trans.). West Stockbridge, MA: Lindisfarne Press. (Original work published 1963)

Schwaller de Lubicz, R. A. (1985a). *Esoterism and symbol* (A. VandenBroeck & G. VandenBroeck, Trans.). New York, NY: Inner Traditions International. (Original work published 1960)

Schwaller de Lubicz, R. A. (1985b). *The Egyptian miracle: An introduction to the wisdom of the temple* (A. VandenBroeck & G. VandenBroeck, Trans.). New York, NY: Inner Traditions International. (Original work published 1963)

Schwaller de Lubicz, R. A. (1988a). *Sacred science: The king of pharaonic theocracy* (A. VandenBroeck & G. VandenBroeck). Rochester, VT: Inner Traditions International. (Original work published 1961)

Schwaller de Lubicz, R. A. (1998b). *The temple of man: Apet of the South at Luxor* (2 vols.) (R. Lawlor & D. Lawlor, Trans.). Rochester, VT: Inner Traditions. (Original work published 1957)

Schwaller de Lubicz, R. A., & Lamy, L. (1977). *The temple in man: The secrets of ancient Egypt* (R. Lawlor & D. Lawlor, Trans.). New York, NY: Autumn Press. (Original work published 1949)

Schweizer, A. (2010). *The sungod's journey through the netherworld: Reading the ancient Egyptian Amduat* (D. Lorton, Ed.). Ithaca, NY: Cornell University Press. (Original work published 1994)

Science. (2011). In *Oxford advanced American dictionary*. Retrieved from http://oaadonline.oxfordlearnersdictionaries.com/dictionary/science

Shaw, I. (2003). *The Oxford history of ancient Egypt* (new ed.). New York, NY: Oxford University Press.

Sheldrake, R. (1987). Part I: Mind, memory, and archetype: Morphic resonance and the collective unconscious. *Psychological Perspectives, 18*(1), 19–25.

Sheldrake, R. (2009). *Morphic resonance: The nature of formative causation*. Rochester, VT: Park Street Press.

Sheldrake, R. (2012). *Science set free: 10 paths to new discovery*. New York, NY: Chopra Books.

Siegel, B. S. (1986). *Love, medicine, and miracles: Lessons learned about self-healing from a surgeon's experience with exceptional patients*. New York, NY: Harper.

Snow, D. (2010). *Archaeology of Native North America*. Boston, MA: Prentice Hall.

Sorell, T. (2000). *Descartes: A very short introduction*. New York, NY: Oxford University Press.

Spence, L. (1990). *Ancient Egyptian myths and legends*. New York: Dover Publications.

Steiner, R. (1911). *The education of children from the standpoint of theosophy* (M. Gysi, Ed.). Chicago, IL: Rajput Press.

Steiner, R. (1971). *Egyptian myths and mysteries: Twelve lectures, Leipzig, September 2–14, 1908* (N. MacBeth, Trans.). New York, NY: Anthroposophic Press. (Original work published 1911)

Steiner, R. (1994). *Theosophy: An introduction to the spiritual processes in human life and in the cosmos*. Hudson, NY: Anthroposophic Press.

Steiner, R. (1998). *Art as spiritual activity: Rudolf Steiner's contribution to the visual arts* (M. Howard, Ed.). Hudson, NY: Anthroposophic Press.

Stocks, Denys A. (2003). *Experiments in Egyptian archaeology: Stoneworking technology in Ancient Egypt*. London, England: Routledge.

Strathern, P. (2007). *Napoleon in Egypt*. New York, NY: Bantam Books.

Talbot, M. (1991). *The holographic universe*. New York, NY: HarperCollins.

Talbot, M. (1992). *Mysticism and the new physics*. London, England: Arkana.

Tarnas, R. (2006). *Cosmos and psyche: Intimations of a new world view*. New York, NY: Viking.

Tart, C. T. (2009). *The end of materialism: How evidence of the paranormal is bringing science and spirit together*. Oakland, CA: Noetic Books/New Harbinger.

Tingley, K. A. W. (1992). *The Gods await*. Pasadena, CA: Theosophical University Press.

Troward, T. (1904). *The Edinburgh and Doré lectures on mental science*. Marina Del Rey, CA: DeVorss.
Troward, T. (1909). *The Doré lectures*. London, England: Stead.
Troward, T. (1991). *The creative process in the individual*. Marina del Rey, CA: DeVorss.
VandenBroeck, A. (1987). *Al-Kemi: Hermetic, occult, political, and private aspects of R. A. Schwaller de Lubicz*. Hudson, NY: Lindisfarne Press.
Varvoglis, M. (2009). What is psi? What isn't? Retrieved from http://archived.parapsych.org/what_is_psi_varvoglis.htm
von Franz, M.-L. (1980). *Alchemy: An introduction to the symbolism and the psychology*. Toronto, Canada: Inner City Books.
von Franz, M.-L. (1992). *Psyche and matter*. Boston, MA: Shambhala.
Wallace, B. A. (2000). *The taboo of subjectivity: Toward a new science of consciousness*. New York, NY: Oxford University Press.
Weberman, D. (2000). A new defense of Gadamer's hermeneutics. *Philosophy and Phenomenological Research, 60*(1), 45–65. http://dx.doi.org/10.2307/2653427
Wehr, G., & Lauer, H. E. (2002). *Jung and Steiner: The birth of a new psychology*. Great Barrington, MA: Anthroposophic Press.
West, J. A. (1993). *Serpent in the sky: The high wisdom of ancient Egypt*. Wheaton, IL: Quest Books.
White, J. E. M. (1970). *Ancient Egypt: Its culture and history*. Mineola, NY: Dover.
Whitney, M. (Director/Producer), & Whitney, M. (Producer). (1986). *Matter of heart* [Motion picture]. USA: Horizon.
Wikman, M. (2004). *Pregnant darkness: Alchemy and the rebirth of consciousness*. Berwick, ME: Nicolas-Hays.
Wilber, K. (2001a). Preface. In K. Wilber (Ed.), *Quantum questions: Mystical writings of the world's great physicists* (pp. xi–xii). Boston, MA: Shambhala.
Wilber, K. (Ed.). (2001b). *Quantum questions: Mystical writings of the world's great physicists*. Boston, MA: Shambhala.
Wilson, C. (1973). *The occult: A history*. New York, NY: Vintage Books.
Wolf, F. A. (1989). *Taking the quantum leap: The new physics for nonscientists*. New York, NY: HarperPerennial.
Wolf, F. A. (1996a). Quantum rules of the universe. In R. E. Dicarlo (Ed.), *Towards a new world view: Conversations at the leading edge* (pp. 58–64). Erie, PA: Epic Publishing.
Wolf, F. A. (1996b). *The spiritual universe: How quantum physics proves the existence of the soul*. New York, NY: Simon.
Woods, R. (2011). *Meister Eckhart: Master of mystics*. London, England: Continuum.
Yourgrau, P. (2005). *A world without time: The forgotten legacy of Gödel and Einstein*. New York, NY: Basic Books.
Zabriskie, B. (2004). Imagination as laboratory. *Journal of Analytical Psychology, 49*(2), 235–242. http://dx.doi.org/10.1111/j.1465-5922.2004.00455.x
Zagorin, P. (1998). *Francis Bacon*. Princeton, NJ: Princeton University Press.

INDEX